A WEIGHT OFF MY MIND

My Life and the Story of
Weight Watchers

A WEIGHT OFF MY MIND

My Life and the Story of Weight Watchers

Bernice Weston

Macdonald

A Macdonald Book

First published in Great Britain in 1991 by
Macdonald & Co (Publishers) Ltd
London & Sydney

British Library Cataloguing-in-Publication Data
Weston, Bernice
A weight off my mind.
I. Title
920

ISBN 0 356 20168 6

Typeset by Leaper & Gard Ltd, Bristol
Printed and bound in Great Britain by
BPCC Hazell Books
Aylesbury, Bucks, England.
Member of BPCC Ltd.

Macdonald & Co (Publishers) Ltd
165 Great Dover Street
London SE1 4YA
A member of Maxwell Macmillan Publishing Corporation

To my children Alesia, Graeme and Douglas Weston, who paid dearly for Weight Watchers. They survived admirably and have been a source of great pride to me. I dedicate this book to them with deep gratitude and much love.

ACKNOWLEDGEMENTS

This book has seemed like the work of a lifetime; indeed, it has taken several years to write. Many people have contributed to the various stages of the book's creation and I extend to all of them my grateful thanks. In particular, I would like to express my gratitude to all my Weight Watchers' supervisors, lecturers, clerks and weighers to whom this book is a tribute — a celebration of the power of people to change major aspects of their lives beneficially for themselves, their family and their community. Also to the members of Weight Watchers: women, children, teenagers and men who believed and continue to believe in the commonsense 'hands on' approach that has made Weight Watchers such an enviable success and so much a part of current British folklore.

Thanks are also due to: Hugh Douglas, Barbara Hardwick, Margaret Mears, Gillian Rimmer, Lee Rodwell and Rowena Webb who helped bring from my locked stores of memory the story I tell today; Virginia Levin, godmother extraordinaire, who at eighty-two writes better than ever I could, for her excellent comments and research, as well as her 'high-kicks' in testing the WiseWeighs exercises; Miriam Rothschild, aged eighty-four, who through her example taught me the value of continuous devotion to work and lifted me off the floor when it seemed this book would never be published; my sister Diana Kirschenbaum who early in life sacrificed much that was rightfully hers to direct my energies into happy and creative accomplishments; Patricia Hatry, friend, confidante, playmate and confrère who stood by me with advice and assistance over many long years and who has proven that with proper exercise and activity the years *can* be pushed back; Douglas Weston, eldest son who read, reread and helped to fashion parts of my story that were painful to us both, so that the truth might be told — more fairly — and of course to Richard Weston, who shared my dream and helped make it happen — and who still brings forth glorious memories as well as unresolved despair. His diet for living created a banquet for many, in which every dish was topped with extravagance — too rich for some, but then for him life was always a one-man fireworks display.

'I think it could be plausibly argued that changes of diet are more important than changes of dynasty or even of religion.'

The Road to Wigan Pier
George Orwell, 1937

CONTENTS

FOREWORD

I first met Bernice Weston when she glowed her way into my office at the *Financial Times*, for which I wrote on many subjects, including business.

'Glowed' was the only word for Bernice. Her hair, her skin, her eyes, even her voice all glowed. One felt the warmth-and-energy halo she carried. Her husband, Richard, was with her. The opposite of the talkative, vital and restless Bernice, there was nevertheless such an obvious if invisible link between them — one felt that, alone, they would be unable to keep their hands off each other.

She had recently become a Weight Watchers success story in America and, fired with faith and her usual enthusiasm, had bought the rights to run the business in Britain. She was about to start classes near her Berkshire home. Richard, as a lawyer, had seen to all the formal and business affairs.

Bernice was really the only asset apart from the proven system of eating in America, but one realised at once what an asset she was. I knew she would do what she planned and would do it well. That she did so, very successfully, is history.

The one thing I couldn't believe was that this slim, vital being had ever been fat and sluggish as she described. Oh yes, she showed me the photographs and I had to believe, but it wasn't easy.

Since then, our paths have crossed many times. There have been short periods of slippage and Bernice has gained a few pounds here and there, but very few. Normally, she eats wisely — by instinct as well as by the habit of many years, and the vitality remains as glowing as on that day so many years ago.

She's a complex character. Very intelligent and caring, she is a keen observer of national and world politics and a sharp critic of both. She is a loving mother — I believe she may also be a good mother but lost touch with her children when they were very young and, surely, only children can say whether a mother is good or not. But loving she is. She is a mixture of natural and sophisticated, of driving ambition and of periodic contentment. She has loved men without ever losing her individuality, being both clinging and loving at the same time as also independent and go-getting. She thinks nothing of dashing halfway across the world when her loved ones need her, and has done it many times.

She is fiercely Jewish, and many of her caring qualities obviously stem from her racial and religious background. She loves to get people together in groups so that everyone can help each other and, in so doing, ultimately help themselves. Group therapy was the basis of Weight Watchers but Bernice feels that groups can do more than share slimming problems. They can share others — financial, emotional, bereavement: anything.

She is right, of course. Just sharing helps, even if one comes only slowly and painfully to being able to talk about oneself in any context. Bernice's own powerful ability to talk, talk, talk in no way seems to lessen her ability to listen and to care and to advise with basic common sense.

When she talks, listen. When she writes, read.

Sheila Black

PREFACE

A funny thing happened to me in the course of writing this autobiography: I gained weight again and developed a weight problem I couldn't lick by my usual tried and tested methods.

Previously Weight Watchers had been a watershed in my life, helping me to lose weight successfully for the first time and to maintain that weight loss for twenty years — no mean feat. Having gone on to found Weight Watchers in Great Britain, I had helped one and a half million people learn how to eat sensibly and lose weight through a system that gave them dietary knowledge, and later support in maintaining their weight loss and leading a normal healthy life. Worldwide, Weight Watchers had helped almost 13 million people achieve the satisfaction of solving their weight problems.

But I seemed unable to do the same for myself the second time around.

Looking back in order to write these memoirs — opening doors on my life which I had shut and bolted in self-preservation, remembering parts which had been painful and which I would have liked to relive differently — shook me seriously, and the weight problems I'd thought were behind me for good became a serious worry once more. The trouble was compounded by a fall downstairs at my office in Ashton, Northamptonshire, which hospitalized me with a hairline fracture of the spine and made it impossible for me to exercise or even take serious walks for more than six months. A similar accident when I was eleven had triggered my original weight gain as a girl; now I was putting on pounds again, unable to stop myself.

I am a superstitious person and it seemed to me, in my weakened state after the accident, that I was being influenced once more by two powerful characters who had formed my earlier attitudes to food — my 'overcaring' mother who fed her family to the point of obesity and, more tragically, my husband Richard. Larger than life in every sense, he was a gifted, sensitive, vulnerable man whose overpowering love of food and antipathy towards the business of dieting dominated and eventually destroyed our business, shook our marriage and endangered his life.

I did not return to my highest lifetime weight but I did put on a stone (far too much for my height of 5 feet 2 inches). My figure and facial outlines changed and my self-confidence was shaken. I found it difficult this time just to return to class and start again as thousands of Weight Watchers have done successfully over the years. Instead, building on what I had learned with (and because of) Weight Watchers, I began to experiment on myself and to find my own personal holistic way to weight loss, vitality and enhanced health.

I felt very strongly that I needed something that was missing from Weight Watchers: exercise. I was beginning to find a new way to slenderness and fitness. I began to walk, slowly at first, then more rapidly — but regularly — so that it became a part of my everyday lifestyle. I began to climb stairs wherever I could find them, to exercise on the floor, on chairs, on buses, on trains, even at my desk — wherever I was, I just kept moving.

I had to do it my way and create my own diet and exercise banks, balancing what I ate against the energy I expended. I had to bank on myself, become my own diet bank manager — and thus was born my new Bank Balance Diet.

To balance the books of good health, however, I needed — and wanted — company and support, yet gyms and health clubs were for me both distracting and very lonely. I needed the support of others to help me stick to a regime which suited me and allow me the luxury of sharing and testing my new theories on diet and exercise with similarly afflicted weight gainers. My research and ideas came together in a new philosophy of diet and exercise: Wise-Weighs.

Soon my friends and I were talking about Chairobics, Stairobics, Floorobics, Cama(Spanish for bed)robics, and Trim-nastics. It didn't matter what we called it: we found that by careful planning and dogged determination we could make exercise a regular counterbalance to the number of calories we ate every day — resulting in weight maintenance, or a way of debiting them — resulting in weight loss.

The group with which I started to exercise developed further to adapt to other transitional crises which members were experiencing in their own lives. Soon I decided to adopt a new concept of total care to be called 'Women in Transition' or the WIT of WiseWeighs, putting advice on diet and exercise into the broadest possible context within the general well-being of the individual.

Now, in 1991, WiseWeighs is poised to enter Britain just as Weight Watchers was in 1967. The journey through these years is the story of my adult life. It has taken me from the all-American heart of Jewish Brooklyn to the gentlest of villages in the part of England known as 'the Shires'. It has been an adventure full of exhilarating experiences, a journey over many bumpy roads, not easy, but packed full of living. It has been shared by so many people — family, friends, colleagues, and the millions of fellow women and men who worked with me, and were a part of Weight Watchers. It has taken me from America to England, around the world and back again to my new self in Britain, a long way from my parents' house in Brooklyn, where I first developed a 'weight on my mind'.

CHAPTER ONE

'When times are bad — you should eat good.'
Mrs Celia Turkewitz

'If I had my life to live over, I'd live it over a grocery store' —
so the popular vaudeville song goes, and so it was for me
and in that marvellous, no-class with lots-of-class neighbourhood in Brooklyn where I was born. I grew up, the
local grocer's daughter, surrounded by warmth, food,
togetherness, food — and yet more food.

It never struck me that I was anything but over-privi-
leged! While the late 1930s were lean times for new Jewish
immigrants to New York, our home was never short of what
we were taught were the essentials of life. My parents,
having come from Pinsk on the Russian-Polish border in
the year 1928, lost all they had in the Wall Street Crash.
They were forced to open a small shop selling foodstuffs.
Living just over the store, or next door, made it easy for
them to establish a prima facie case as good parents; as my
mother often said, 'When times are bad — you should eat
good.' This philosophy she carried through life, and from it
resulted a fat husband and three fat children.

We were fed not only on demand, but on special occasions. Special occasions happened for us every day and took
the form of three four-course meals, a malted milk with
extra malt and an egg for nourishment, bread and jam, lox
(smoked salmon), cream cheese and a pickle 'to fight
disease'. Cookies or biscuits were for scraped knees, apple
pie for when the teacher told you off, chocolate for when
you could or couldn't go to the movies, anything you

wanted from the store (with extra butter) when a guest arrived. Plus however much extra you could put away on the weekend and holidays!

Being from Brooklyn is like being a Hungarian — it's a profession. And the tools of our profession came wrapped in chicken fat. The streets of Brooklyn, even today, are a symphony of smells, a cacophony of sounds selling pizza, hot dogs, egg rolls, ice cream, frozen custard, hamburgers, chestnuts, chick peas and fried shrimp on a stick.

Only in my day everything that came on a stick had to be kosher, and what is more the names of the purveyors of these joys had to *sound* kosher. There was Shmulka Bernstein's salami, Yonah Schimmel's knishes, Eisenberg's egg-creams and Mother's gefilte fish. For those who 'strayed' or wanted to declare their independence, there was always the Chinese restaurant. Here happy Chinese waiters always obliged those like me who lost their nerve at the last minute; to us they served a lettuce and tomato sandwich on well-done toast, or in the Brooklyn vernacular: 'An L-T-Down, Cremated'.

Food meant love and there was no shortage of second helpings. Among our neighbours were immigrants who had come from many lands. They brought with them the only treasures they could carry, in many cases recipes and little else. But what treasures they were. A little girl walking happily amidst all the rich and diverse aromas coming from different kitchen windows, and being offered tastes of this and tastes of that, could develop a real sense of security and expect only good things from people forever after.

Mamma taught us to cross over the street and say 'hello' to anyone we knew; and we always received a 'hello, how are you' and sometimes a taste of something in return. It was a magic world where everyone was a foreigner yet a one hundred per cent 'Yankee' at the same time. Hardly any of the adults spoke English properly except the chemist who was looked upon as the official translator of any English letter or official-looking document. There was of course Mr

Blackbeer, our tailor, who came from Liverpool and spoke the King's English. For years he was ostracised: 'Only a spy could speak such good English,' we thought. Years later when I opened my first Weight Watchers class in Liverpool, I was astounded to discover that not all Liverpudlians were grammarians — so 'stuck up' did our English tailor appear, just because he could speak English grammatically and pronounce all his w's and th's.

We talked of food constantly; it was part of every aspect of our lives. My mother rose early to begin baking and preparing, determined that because she worked full-time in the store, some twelve hours a day, her children would still have meals on time and 'not be without'. Every Jewish holiday became associated with food; even a day of fasting became a painless experience, because you could plan what you would eat before the fast, which would sustain you through it, and then of course you could eat gloriously afterwards. The emphasis on food did not take away from the religiosity of the occasion. Could a Jewish God possibly be put off if one enjoyed a good meal as well?

My mother also had a very real conviction that fat children were less likely to develop TB or contract any serious illness. This was (and unfortunately still is) quite a commonly held belief. It was as if people believed that diseases like cancer and tuberculosis took longer to 'get to you' if you had a layer of fat as protection. Fat meant healthy. A good mother was one who raised a fat child.

There is a saying that chicken soup is the Jewish penicillin; certainly this was totally accepted as a maxim in our neighbourhood where no illness was known to exist that could not be tackled and treated with food. 'A sick person, you ask. A healthy person, you just give' — how often did I hear my mother say this?

It was not only our particular neighbourhood which was food-orientated. New York is full of different ghettos which have established their individual identities by the smell of their cooking. There are entire streets which smell only of bread and pickled herring. The German quarter seems to have a cloud of sauerkraut steam constantly hovering above it; the Viennese walk to and from work, either finishing or just starting an eclair; while the Hungarians and Romanians vie as to who can put more paprika into a dish. I remember a friend saying that in New York you follow your nose to a particular neighbourhood rather than looking at street signs. Whatever the ethnic group, whatever the country of origin, food was primarily a comforter and a reassurer.

I remember as a young child there was great excitement at an incident which had taken place on the Lower East Side — then the home of Jewish pushcart peddlers. There was a bottom pincher loose in the neighbourhood; a man who went around making a nuisance of himself by disturbing elderly and religious women. The women finally organized a vigilante team and when he was caught they hounded him into a small alleyway, surrounding him in a circle and began hitting him with their handbags, swinging wildly with feathered and unfeathered chickens and bags of groceries. They then made him put on his skull cap and confess his sins before all and sundry onlookers. He looked such a picture of abject misery that the women soon began to feel sorry for him and in typical fashion were soon feeding him to make him feel better. This impressed upon me the power of food to ameliorate any situation, however bizarre.

It used to be a running joke in our family to try to get Mamma to sit down. She never did because she was always serving. She didn't realise that we needed her and her companionship more than we needed her food. She could never join us at table because she was always dishing out a second helping, or a third, or preparing for the next course. Because of this I promised myself that I would not be a 'server' to my children; that I would be a sharer and, unlike my mother, sit down with them at mealtimes because second helpings would not be part of my family regime. Yet when I am tired and low in spirits I find myself losing control and falling back into the old habit of serving and filling them up with food, instead of giving them portions of time with me. It is hard work totally to blot out a deeply engrained pattern from one's life, but important to understand how formative are such childhood habits.

I sincerely believed, because of my upbringing, that the only time one should leave a dinner table was when one felt uncomfortable — or 'stuffed'. I did not know that there were places in the world where people left merely because they had had enough, rather than because they could not eat any more.

If food was a way of expressing love in our home, it was also a way of bribing us to study. School and learning was another form of nourishment, as desirable as a well-prepared dish. To people with an immigrant mentality, food was reassurance as well as reward, but *education* — ah, education meant a *future*. With an education you had a 'needle in your hand' that you could take anywhere. For people who had grown up amidst pogroms and political upheaval, it was essential to provide their children with an inheritance of learning and culture that could never be taken away. So reading and studying were rewarded with a treasure trove of toffee and other fattening treats.

The family fridge was the treasure house, each shelf reserved for a particular child. For my brother Hy the medical student who studied into the morning hours, the top shelf was set aside to be filled with cheese, sausages, pickled this and pickled that — the hard stuff, to fortify him through his night-time romance with Science. My sister 'Dina-Leh' or Diana, 'the chubby one' as she was lovingly called, was the soft-ware specialist: ice cream, sherbets, fudge toppings, and anything between and below whipped cream toppings.

As the baby, I was allowed and encouraged to develop more catholic tastes. These came in the form of the pasta, salami and sauces which our Catholic Italian landlady, Mrs

Carlo, prepared. She had agreed before I was born that she and the Carlo clan would 'mind me', and she kept her word. While my mother worked from 6 a.m. to midnight, seven days a week, in the store with my father, Mrs Carlo and her numerous offspring would stuff me with all the magical recipes which begin with garlic paste, tomatoes, and pasta with everything. To this very day when I feel really low or out of sorts, there is nothing more right or more uplifting than a plate of spaghetti, with a Neapolitan melody playing softly in the background.

My mother and father came to America in 1928. They brought two small children — one an infant — my father's brother, and, like The Owl, 'plenty of money' to begin their new life. My father had been successful at an early age in the arbitrage business in Russia. He was strong, bright and full of optimism.

Within a year the money was lost in the Wall Street Crash. My mother, whose family was well-to-do, professional, and highly respected in Pinsk, was ashamed to return in their impoverished state. Pinsk had been the birthplace of Golda Meir and the boyhood playing grounds of Chaim Weitzmann and other well-known Zionist leaders. She and my father decided to remain for a while — although they were both unhappy in this strange new land. They hoped quickly to regain enough capital to go home other than as paupers. This decision proved a fateful one. My mother's entire family — mother, five sisters, two brothers, their wives and children, all her relatives — were later killed in the early forties when the 'final solution' of the Germans destroyed within a matter of days the entire Jewish population in Pinsk. I feel that my mother's capacity for joy died when she discovered the facts of her family's deaths immediately after the war.

She and Poppa borrowed enough money to buy a grocery store in Brooklyn, New York, and there they worked, seven days a week, sometimes ten to twelve hours at a stretch, always courteous, always kind, never familiar.

Turkewitz's grocery store, which furnished Morris and
Celia Turkewitz with a livelihood and assuaged the hunger
of my brother, sister and me, was also the local courthouse
and a political arena. We three children found a marvellous
fountain at which to drink up an understanding of different
kinds of people and to hear them out. My father was a
dedicated Labor—Zionist with strong socialist leanings
(until he entered the real estate world and learned about
property taxes). He educated himself not only in the business world, but in the world of music and song. He sang
beautifully and often. When he lost all his wealth in the
Wall Street Crash, speaking little English and having no
trade, he had no choice but to take his young wife and
babes into what he always considered his 'prison' — a small
grocery store, with small profits and small-minded
customers. But issues were important to him and he read
his Jewish newspaper from cover to cover and engaged
every customer in some political or philosophical argument
or another.

Yet, above all he believed and guided us to believe, in a
life of service inherited from his own dedicated and highly
philanthropic mother.

He taught us that the needs of the community or of a
particular neighbour were always very much our business
too. Each morning he would rise, take in the cases of
bottled milk left outside and start to sweep the sidewalk in
front of his store. Next he would move to the next store
front, and the next, and the next. Our customers would
arrive and wait. Soon their wails for help would reach my
mother upstairs. 'Mrs Turkewitz, help, my husband has to
go to work. I need milk and I can't give him his breakfast
because your husband has to clean the whole world.' 'Mr
Turkewitz, stop already, stop! Give someone else a chance.
This is the land of opportunity — everyone has the opportunity to sweep his own shop front.' 'Hurry up, or I'll shop
by Rubenstein.'

It never dawned on my father that the dirt across the

street was not his problem, nor that cleaning the other side of the street was positively bad for his business. What did matter was that the streets should be clean for the children to pass through on their way to school, and that with a clean neighbourhood, local people would keep their pride and self-respect.

If an old person seemed confused, we were sent from our house to see them home; if a child was injured and the mother not available, we were sent to take him for his stitches; if there was an argument among neighbours, we settled it at the back of the store. Most customers paid their bills when they could, even though Poppa had difficulty paying his own on time. He was gentle, soft spoken and full of fun, except when there was a political argument: this did not end until someone walked out, slammed the door, and a window pane fell out.

Mamma was the keeper of secrets, everyone's confidante. She hated gossip and taught us early in life just how dangerous tale bearing could be. I truly believe that without her teaching I could never have worked with the 2,000-odd Weight Watchers lecturers, clerks, weighers and other female staff and made a go of it; if I hadn't learnt how to prevent tittle-tattle or stop it dead, the largely female workforce could not have dealt with the business in hand.

As children we were allowed to stay in the store only on condition that we repeated nothing we heard and never, never criticised a customer, no matter how angry they made us or how unfairly we thought they treated our folks. Once again, in my Weight Watchers experience I went on to teach everyone who worked for us that our prime job was to serve the little fat lady who came for the first or the sixteenth time to a class for help: it was our creed that she was more important, more right, than anyone else.

When our first professional adviser drew up an organizational chart putting my husband and myself at the top as Founder-Directors, I had her re-draft the entire chart and put me and my associates at the bottom, holding up and supporting the 'member', who was always on top and whose interest always came first.

I market tested as my folks did, not through market research organizations testing fifty 'representative' families, but by going out on the streets with our prospective product or to a class and letting my members taste and sample ... and decide, just as my father would 'give taste with a spoon' to a customer before he took in a new line. It worked! We sold what our members really wanted, not what an advertising man advised that they wanted.

When our dog Skippy ran out of the house without a lead and we were summoned to court with a risk of having him taken away, Harry the postman told all, and the community organized itself. My father was taken off to join the local Democrats Political Club so that the District Leader might use his influence with the Judge to buy us a 'suspended sentence'. From that moment on I was a loyal Democrats party worker, carrying nominating petitions and 'getting out the vote'. It didn't seem wrong to me at the age of six to save a dog by giving justice a nudge, and even today I wonder how else immigrants with no power and no pull could protect their rights, help obtain equal opportunities for their children or protect their puppy dogs without community efforts, even ones as questionable as this.

Many years later, when I was involved in local New York City politics and joined groups devoted to 'throwing the rascals out', I found that even those rascals had something to say for themselves; many of them started with a real, if perhaps misguided, desire to help people. I learned not to condemn easily nor to judge too quickly.

Again, with the Weight Watchers member who cheated or gained weight, condemnation was out of the question and listening became both an art and the foundation of everything we tried to do in the field of weight loss.

I was in danger of becoming fat throughout my childhood but weight did not become a problem for me until my eleventh year. I broke my leg at the beginning of the summer whilst at a children's vacation camp and was taken back to a hot, lonely city to sweat out a long New York summer. Everyone felt sorry for me and brought me ice-cream sodas, ice-cream sundaes, ice-cream Tuesdays and double chocolate milk shakes. I would average about one or two of each of these in a day as I sat reading comics, history and Shakespeare, surrounded by layers of hot fudge, melted marshmallow, honeyed walnuts and three scoops of ice cream at any one time. My leg got better but my figure worsened. By summer's end I had blossomed and bloomed into a 'zoftic', well-read and well-rounded eleven-stone eleven year old.

Because I was fat I took the easy way out: I became a tom-boy. I was a great athlete, the equal of any boy on the baseball diamond or the basketball court, but a complete washout at parties. I was immensely insecure with my femininity. At just the age when I should have been blossoming, I became aggressively tomboyish. Luckily I had many boys among my friends, but I found it easier to be accepted as one of them, not as a girl or, more important, a prospective date.

For a while I was known as 'Slugger Turk' because I once 'slugged' a boy who tried to kiss me, and that name lasted throughout my mid-teens. It was easier to fall into that role and be droll and a load of laughs. I roller-skated to school, did bicycle tricks, won handball championships and ran fifty-yard races. I was always the clown with a fund of anec-dotes and funny stories, and always playing the clown's role in the school plays, never those puny, silly romantic leads. When I played baseball it was to win, and I would chase and attack any girl who didn't run fast enough around the bases. I played hard — none of that helpless, defenceless female role for me.

Strangely enough everyone, especially my family, thought that I was perfectly happy and worried not at all about their fat, unfeminine daughter. My father used to brag, in fact, that one could have chopped wood on my bottom, so round, so firm, so resilient was his plump little daughter.

But I loved to dance and parties, to which you had to be invited, were the usual place to dance socially. Many was the time I walked off a playing field, arm in arm with a boy I liked, only to have him disengage himself while he asked a silly wisp of a girl to be his date that night. Still, there was always Solly, my childhood sweetheart. He danced like a dream and was understanding and loyal as well. He wasn't sought after either, so we would go to the movies on 'dish' night — when pieces of crockery were given away as an incentive to the audience — and see the old Fred Astaire and Ginger Rogers films over and over again until we had memorised all the routines. Then we would take tons of hamburgers and orange squash on to a roof top and dance out the routines and all our fantasies.

I think the joy of dancing and the pleasure of knowing that we did it well helped me overcome the real hurt and those gnawing doubts about myself which pretty well took up most of my adolescent years. Difficult as adolescence can be for anyone, it was made very much more difficult for me, as it always is for fat youngsters, because I could not accept myself the way I was, yet couldn't find a solution to my problem appearance.

As a student I was conscientious and hard-working, but I used my success as another protective shield. I always entered a bus showing off my school books or some esoteric novel. I hoped people would look at me and think, 'Well, she may not be a beauty, but at least she's brainy'. I was an attention-seeker, a non-stop talker and joke-teller, but behind my extrovert craziness I was also introspective and constantly seeking ways of developing compensatory skills to offset my fatness. So on the outside I was the typical jolly fat person whom everyone would have described then as a happy, sturdy (sturdy here was fat turned solid), normal girl. Nobody for a moment realized or was allowed to realize that I minded being fat; they thought it was just part of being Bernice.

At home and in our neighbourhood there was no stigma attached to being overweight; almost everyone was. But at Winthrop Junior High School, I began to meet and observe another type of student — real middle-class kids whose parents spoke English and went out for dinner, and whose mothers dressed smartly, wore perfume and were slim. It was true that my mother wasn't fat but she was perpetually concealed in an apron, cooking or serving.

It was at Winthrop Junior School that I first had learned the power that slim people have over fat ones. I saw that there was a natural authority that came with thinness, and that it was much easier to be self-assertive if one liked the way one looked.

One day my friend Sarah's mother came to school to confront one of our teachers who was both fat and a bully. I was amazed. To my mother, as to all the mothers in our neighbourhood, respect for teachers was absolute. A teacher could do no wrong. But into this repository of complete authority came Sarah's mother — thin and elegant, high heels clicking as she came down the hall. She opened the door and motioned the teacher to join her, and as she talked I watched our fat bullying teacher completely humble herself before this self-assured thin woman. Thin power had triumphed once again, and I was both witness and convert.

By the time I entered junior high school I had developed a reputation that frightened most teachers to death. I was the class jester, the outrageous tomboy bubbling over with surplus energy — and this energy spelled trouble for law and order. When Miss Rose Schor, my English teacher, saw my reports, she paled at the prospect of my entering her class — but she did not balk from taking me in hand in just the right way. She kept me busy doing constructive things, working overtime at school and at home; it was she who encouraged me to read history and biography for the first time and put me into the school debating society; she encouraged me to write stories and to right wrongs, both political and social. I didn't realise it at the time but she was channelling that excess energy. I joined the school newspaper and convinced myself that I would be a great journalist. When I became editor of the school newspaper, I began visiting those far-off places in Manhattan that meant culture, charm and panache, and all of them filled with thin, elegant-looking people. It seemed to be summed up in one phrase: 'If you want to be in, you've got to be thin.'

By the time I entered high school I began to have other boyfriends; boys who respected me for my abilities. With one of them, Max Brandt, I began covering stories for a reporter on the *New York Herald Tribune.* He would give us free passes for all the important sporting events and we would supply him with the story for a fee of $5 to cover 'expenses' — extra food and malts, which we ate ravenously while we watched these important events. This arrangement worked marvellously well until the day that Doris Hart, who had never been beaten in an indoor tennis match, took on an unknown at the Women's Indoor Tennis Championship at Madison Square Gardens. Max and I were supposed to cover the story for the reporter, but we were talked into leaving early to catch a smashing film at Radio City Music Hall instead. We wrote our story about Doris Hart's normal victory, cabled it in and left before the famous upset of that night. The story was printed as we wrote it and our journalist boss got the sack while we lost our passes. Because of that incident I don't think I shall ever leave any event early. Because of that incident I learned an important lesson: if you take on a job, do it well, stay on and finish it.

I soon learned how to join the system instead of fighting it. I needed the attention I received for doing constructive and creative work. I was afraid of audiences so I cured myself by joining the debating society and forcing myself to speak before huge and varied audiences. I became the school leader and a teenage star. I was voted The Girl Most Likely to Succeed and The Girl Most Likely to Burn Out

Before She Is 21. I was outwardly sophisticated and appeared totally sure of myself, but inwardly I became more insecure.

I was now travelling out of the neighbourhood more frequently. Up until then much of my life had begun, continued and ended in Brooklyn, from whence all good things came. Now my interests and my scope were widening and a big, sophisticated, thin world spread out before me. What do girls do when they are ambitious, bright, and want to enter a world where there is glamour and where exciting things happen? They either enter the world of fashion or the theatre or a profession.

As a child Brooklyn society was fine by me, but as I matured I wanted to be at the centre of things. Because I accepted that I wouldn't make my way into the worlds of fashion or theatre in a size 16, I plotted my way out of my comfortable surroundings and entered a new world by becoming a recruit to a profession not often open to women. I decided to go to law school and announced this in my usual precipitate way to all and sundry. My parents were concerned and frightened for me. Why do something so unusual? Why not follow the normal safe way: become a teacher or a fashion buyer, and stay close to home?

Actually they hoped that I would marry young like my sister and my friends who had chosen to settle down early in life, many marrying just after they left high school. But I chose to enter Brooklyn Law School which did much, not only to further my career but also to boost my ego. There were six girls in the class and one hundred and fifty men. How easy it is to be sought after, and to be made to feel attractive, when the odds are so stacked in your favour.

Many of the men in the class were much older. They were reaching pensionable age in their first career and attending school to prepare themselves for a second. In many instances they took a fatherly interest in me and for the first time I began to have people suggest to me that I ought to try doing something about my weight.

I was determined to help out with expenses while my parents carried the burden of paying for my schooling, so I took a part-time job working in the afternoons for the law firm of Hays, Podell, Algase, Crum and Feuer. The five senior partners were a fascinating group. Bartley Crum was a theatrical lawyer, among other things, and our offices were frequently visited by Rita Hayworth, Ali Khan or other film and society types. Another of the partners was a great civil libertarian. Yet another was a man very much involved in international causes and substantial charities. Our clients were important, successful men, and their wives, when they visited the office with them, always appeared elegant and, dear God, were either always thin or else chatted happily to the receptionist about some new diet which was going to make them thin and even more elegant. What was most interesting to me was that the people in this new world seemed to live without placing any emphasis on the role of food in their lives. They liked to do, achieve, see and be seen, and were more interested in where they went to eat, and whom they would see there, than whether the portions were large, or the food well flavoured. This is not to say there were not some amongst them with weight problems, but they were constantly fighting an unrelenting battle to win a slimmer figure and conform to the elegant norm.

I loved working for Bartley Crum. Being a law clerk was about as low as you could get on the rung of success at my law firm. It meant that you carried packages, delivered briefs, served summonses, and frequently went along to meetings with a partner only in case he forgot his pen or needed a pencil sharpened. The joy of working for Bartley Crum was that, whenever I entered a room with him to meet one of his important clients, he always took time to introduce me as 'Bernice Turkewitz, my associate'. At seventeen, being Bartley Crum's associate was no mean thing. I learned from him — something that helped me many years later in my work at Weight Watchers — that if you raise someone working for you to the level of an 'asso-ciate', you find that their level of work, and their devotion to the company and their job, is raised as well. I usually found it more fun anyway to have people working with me than working for me.

I also learned something else while at that firm. I would see bright young men with the highest qualifications enter the office as junior associates and begin working on the most complicated cases. They would work night and day, striving to prepare winning briefs that were worthy of winning. Then the system required that they turn over their painstaking research to more senior members of the firm who would handle the case. The partners and senior asso-ciates took these beautifully prepared briefs for granted and slotted the cases into their schedule, unconcerned. The young researcher and I would sit in the back of the court room, listening to the partner bungling what had been this young man's baby for months on end. Some of the juniors would rush out and throw up in the men's room because they felt so powerless to protect their work and place their own stamp on it. I vowed never to put myself in the same powerless position.

As soon as I finished law school I became my own boss and in every enterprise I have begun since I have chosen to give up 'security' and assume the risk of being self-employed. But I have insisted equally that the people with whom I work be prepared to take the same responsibility for what they do and what they achieve, with the incentive of rewards and credit for their work. This proved to be a key element of the success and extraordinary growth of the Weight Watchers movement in Great Britain. Women who had been failures so long, and who had been kept in the background for so many reasons, were given the limelight and full responsibility not only for their own lives, but for those of others, as well as the success and reputation of an organisation. Among the two thousand or so women who assumed this role working alongside me, I can think of no more than five cases in which I and my fellow lecturers were disappointed.

I enjoyed my job with the law firm and I loved my work at law school. The law is a very exact science and an exacting teacher. From it I learned why it was important to make rules, and how magically people responded when they had rules that were clear and easy to live by.

My life was full of schooling, work, and of course the never-ending round of activities that came with being a political worker and pleader of causes. I joined everything and anything ... law societies, political groups, pressure groups. The young people with whom I mixed were bright, caring and involved. We would sit up through the small hours of the morning arguing about everything, solving few problems but enjoying the discussion nonetheless.

There were high points and low points in my life; most of the high points involved academic, political or career achievements. Most of the low points involved social failures and the inability to think enough of myself really to seek out the people who attracted me most strongly. I 'settled' pretty often for those who were interested in me and very seldom put myself out on a limb for fear of being rejected.

I learned to accommodate my weight but never to accept it. I took short cuts and began to dress more carefully to hide my bulk, wearing high heels that hurt my feet, but made me appear taller and therefore slimmer. I avoided bright colours and dressed in more sombre grey flannel suits and smart dark things. It suited the young lawyer and it pretty well helped to cover the fat young girl inside.

I will never forget, however, one event when I was con- sidered a bright, successful young lawyer, apparently fully content with my life. I shared a flat with three girls. One was the now-famous actress Dyan Cannon and the other two, Barbara DeVorzon and Darlene Jamon, were lovely looking, a swinging model and an artists' representative respectively. I was a size 16 and they were size 6, 8 and 10. We got along famously and there is no doubt that the girls would have given me the clothes off their backs but with all the affection in the world size 8 could never stretch to fit a size 16.

The girls were being constantly rushed off their feet by successful, intelligent and interesting young men, to the 21 Club, the Copacabana ... to all the high-flying 'in' places. Equally they were always protecting me, this intelligent, deep, philosophical and ethical room-mate of theirs, from these wild young men in convertibles. I longed not to be protected but to share part of their sophisticated life.

One afternoon I came home early from the office. It was a hot summer's day and the front door of our flat was open to cause some welcome cross-ventilation. I could hear the girls talking about their planned evening out. One of them suggested that I be asked to join them as a blind date for a friend of one of their boyfriends. 'OK,' said the other, 'but let's introduce her to him sitting down. Maybe he'll listen to her for a while and get to see how bright and nice she is before the full impact of her hits him, when she stands up.'

I knew they meant well and I knew they wouldn't have hurt me for the world, but I also knew that what they were saying was true and, what is more important, I didn't know how I could change things. I did wow them that night, though. I hit them with the sheer force of a personality determined to triumph. It was a fun night but not without its scars.

I began serious dieting when I entered law school; by 'serious' I mean that I was serious when I started, and also serious in that the diets I chose were usually punishing and dangerous both to health and mental equilibrium. For a long time the failure I encountered either during or immediately after a diet affected my life and my personality.

During my last year of law school I was worried enough to seek psychoanalysis and spent long hours and hard-earned cash telling a bright young analyst why I found it difficult to accept my situation. Had it not been for my almost totally happy and supportive family background, I think I would have sustained great damage during this idiotic and punishing period.

The diets weren't without their lighter moments, though, and Lord knows I had enough companions in my sorrowful journey. I remember once having our next-door neighbour race into the house to complain that an earthquake was threatening. Little did he realise it was merely one of my new exercise gimmicks whereby I hit my right and then my left hip and buttock against the wall rhythmically, in the hope that this would diminish the curves and dispel the fat that helped the curves stay curvy.

Fortunately and unfortunately my parents took my struggles with not only a pinch of salt but a plateful of ice cream. They had lived through just such a period with my sister and, after all, hadn't she managed to get married and settle down happily? Why should the same not happen to their baby?

Interestingly enough, the only family ally that I had in the battle to lose weight was my grandmother, Bubby. She was probably the most influential person in my early life. A born matriarch, she had merely to enter a room and people would stand up as if commanded by some unseen force. At 96 she was still very much aware of herself and her appearance. She dressed as befitted a deeply orthodox and religious person, but with panache as well. Her life was devoted to service. She travelled widely (at 90 she took herself off alone on a trip around the world), and everywhere observed the latest fashions as well as the latest in the political, social and religious climates. She was a woman of the world as well as a woman of the spirit and held firmly to very deep religious beliefs. But she was always fun — frequently sought out by my friends for advice on all subjects — and always someone to look up to and to try and pattern oneself upon. She understood that I was not happy with my weight and encouraged me whenever I needed encouragement. It was always helpful for her to say that things were 'God's will' but she believed, as do I, that

God will always accept help from a well-intentioned and well-motivated assistant.

My mother was a marvel as well; although she tempted me and encouraged me to stop dieting, she would join me and aid me constantly in my search for smart clothes for 'the larger frame'. But she did believe quite honestly that I was not fat (at 5 feet $2\frac{1}{2}$ inches ranging between $9\frac{1}{2}$ and 11 stone, approximately 60–70 kg) and still saw me as slight, svelte and without a flaw!

With such a Jewish mother behind you, there is little that you can't accomplish, but a lot that you can't talk about which quietly hurts you and stings deep inside.

It was also during this period that I began my first series of creative ventures. I could never resist a good idea and was constantly hatching new ones to raise funds to augment my skimpy law student's allowance, and those of my friends and associates.

With the benefit of hindsight, I believe that many of those ideas would have been great successes. As a fat girl, though, I lacked that last bit of courage that makes you forsake safety and jump in, prepared to swim until you reach dry land. It was only after I lost weight successfully that I first began to have that extra bit of something, perhaps courage, perhaps self-confidence, which enabled me to take these creative ideas and 'run with them'.

One of the ideas I had at law school was to start an independent film company. It was during one of the encounters I rashly undertook on behalf of that scheme that I met one of America's better known, albeit less than noble, folk heroes. He was an extremely handsome millionaire's son who had become a public figure during the very unfortunate McCarthy era. Although many people did not like his politics, he was still very attractive and much too obnoxious to be ignored. We met by chance and I suppose I was so unlike the usual starlets or models he dated (and possibly because his father wanted him to meet some nice 'balibatish' or respectable girls), he decided to give me a whirl. For me it *was* a whirl: dancing at the Waldorf-Astoria, having dinner at fancy supper clubs, being driven around in chauffeured limousines. It was frequently during these drives that he would engage me in discussions about my size.

'You're such an interesting girl — why don't you do something about your weight?' That was the sort of lead sentence that this brash but frank young man would use in almost all our conversations. Because I did not like his politics I outwardly responded 'What do you know?', but deep down I would have liked to have been able thoroughly to captivate him and then thumb my nose at him, whenever I felt like it. Strangely enough, I did end the relationship. The life he led was attractive but presented too many challenges, too many opportunities for hurt because of my less than perfect figure. It was interesting that the more I advanced in outward sophistication, the less mature I was in my inner emotional life. I was afraid of close relationships which might lead me to care for someone. I felt I couldn't fulfil someone because I could never be an object of desire, and that in turn would lead to hurt — my hurt.

So I took the road that many girls like me frequently take. I became a cause lover and supporter. I threw myself into politics with all the passion I denied myself in my dealings with people.

I became an ardent, almost hysterical, supporter of Adlai Stevenson, a most popular liberal candidate for the Democratic nomination for President of the United States. I worked night and day in the local club-houses for his nomination and as a reward was invited to go to the Chicago Democratic Convention. It meant working even more closely with my idol, and working with even more dedication for his successful nomination.

With a group of other idealistic young people I set out for Chicago in a twenty-year-old car, determined to put everything I had into winning this election away from the bosses and for Adlai.

We patrolled the streets, handed out leaflets, filled in hundreds of nominating petitions, made speeches on street corners, appeared on television shows, invested our own money in pins and posters — and worked around the clock.

One evening as I was returning to campaign headquarters, I entered through the back door, where we stored all our equipment. I could hear two men talking and quickly realised that one of them was Stevenson's principal aide, the other his campaign manager.

'You know,' said one, 'if it weren't for these fat girls I don't know how we'd ever run a political campaign. They're always around to do all the dirty work. Nothing is too much for them, no job too lowly. They never seem to get asked to all the fancy dances or social occasions so they are always available for full-time activity on our behalf. God rue the day when a magic pill can make all women slim. Our candidates couldn't get elected as dog-catchers then.'

They both laughed, and although they were good men, pleasant to work for, and what they said was not meant to cut, it was blindingly, searingly hurtful.

Suddenly all my high-minded ideals and dedicated devotion were brought down to a very common denominator. I was a fat girl whose dedication was devalued, dismissed as compensation for my failure as an attractive human being.

I quietly left headquarters, walked out on to the windy, wet Chicago city streets, and couldn't help adding some very bitter tears to that showery day.

CHAPTER TWO

When I first came to Britain on a visit in the early sixties I had no idea that I would find a husband, family and home there — and of course a career in Weight Watchers. The start of this momentous change was as simple as it was unexpected: a visit to the office of a London lawyer to discuss a copyright matter.

There I first set eyes on the man I was to marry. I did not know at the time, but copyright was not Richard Weston's field. Normally he would have passed me on to someone else in the firm, but he was intrigued by the sound of my voice on the telephone and by the fact that I was a New York lawyer and a girl. He had made up his mind that if I was attractive, he would take me to lunch; otherwise, he would see me briefly and tell me he was busy.

When I walked into his office, my first impression was of a man of 45 or 50, heavy set and heavy jowled, and wearing an unfashionable, old man's suit. Although I didn't know it at the time, Richard was only 25. His mature appearance was caused by his being overweight — probably about 19 stone (121 kilos). He had finished a diet two weeks earlier and had already regained all that he had lost. He was not attractive to me at first, until he moved and spoke. When he moved he became lithe, graceful and most imposing, and when he spoke — ah, when he spoke — his voice was deep, rich and commanding. His whole face and body seemed to take on a different aura. It was like watching an apparently insignificant actor walk on to the stage and then speak, revealing that you are in the presence of a star.

Six minutes after I walked in, Richard had taken me off for lunch; we never returned to the office that day, or to the subject matter of the lawsuit. In the evening, after champagne and dancing, he drove me away in a borrowed Jaguar sports car and proceeded to demonstrate how, when you suddenly step on the brake, you can make the car spin — and spin we did, all around Grosvenor Square.

Then he became romantic, persistently romantic. I was offended and fended him off with the typically Brooklyn Jewish avoidance tactic of talking him deaf, dumb and blind until he took me back to Dolphin Square, where I was staying with my special friends, Ginny and Louis Levin.

That was the start of a hectic, unremitting, cunning, brilliantly tactical wooing such as only Richard Weston could pursue. He began to send me letters and tapes filled with romantic poems and witty observations. He persuaded all his American friends to telephone me and remind me that he still existed. Then he himself turned up in New York on his way to visit friends in Des Moines. He looked dreadful: podgy and tired. Our meeting was not a success — again Richard was persistently 'romantic'; again I rebuffed him — but he arranged through an intermediary for us to meet on his way back to England.

All my friends adored Richard and wanted to entertain him royally, and even I could not escape his spell. When the Waldorf-Astoria restaurant claimed they were fully booked, I called and reserved a table for the Russian Ambassador and Richard carried off the role with enormous panache, foreshadowing Glasnost by a quarter of a century.

He courted me and charmed me with his delicious sense of the absurd — and his daring. One evening during dinner with some influential Ivy League friends he was asked which university he had attended — Oxford or Cambridge — and replied simply, 'I played rugger for both.' Actually, Richard never attended either.

Later that same evening we walked up Fifth Avenue,

Richard dressed in typical English solicitor's suit with stiff shirt collar and cuffs and wearing a summer straw boater, in spite of the fact that it was November and snow was starting to fall. As we passed the famous Steuben Building with its charming fountain and pool, a group of rather drunken rowdy Americans began to taunt him about his dress and lack of overcoat. Richard assured them that Englishmen always acted individually and he personally was so very hot-blooded that seasons meant nothing to him. He needed no overcoat. 'You don't feel the cold?' they asked. 'No,' he replied, 'I don't.' 'Well, how about a swim in this lovely pool?' they said, motioning him to the pool.

Before anyone realized what he was doing, he rolled up his trouser legs, revealing his garters, removed his jacket and jumped into the pool. Taking large swigs of water, he proceeded to pose like a huge fountain statue and began spouting water from his mouth. The drunken Americans were impressed and began to clap wildly, at which point Richard treated them to a brilliant dissertation, inviting Americans to rejoin the Commonwealth, that all was forgiven for 1776. A bus stopped at the corner and the passengers got off and began to cheer. Taxis stopped and the police came to see what was going on, only to discover Richard reciting love poetry to me. Everyone began to urge me to put him out of his misery and be 'his girl'. We ended up in an all-night brasserie eating hot soup and laughing and I was more infatuated with Richard than ever.

However, I had other things on my mind that year of 1962. It was an exciting time for me. I had opened a new office just opposite Carnegie Hall. At first I had planned to specialize in labour relations but soon acquired some interesting theatrical clients and began to work primarily in the field of copyright, in plays, books, music, etc. It was stimulating and exhilarating working with a client-list of playwrights, impresarios, songwriters, musicians, actors and producers — even if at times my income was so low I had to give cha-cha lessons so as to afford the rental of my office and equipment. I helped produce an unsuccessful off-Broadway play entitled *The Jack Ass* and became involved with an equally unsuccessful small budget motion picture. In addition I joined a group who founded the first combined restaurant-theatre-night club in New Jersey and who lost sixty thousand dollars in the first three months. I also had a short spell founding a Geisha Girl School which landed me on television. This too failed. My mother used to say I needed just one success and I would be a hundred per cent ahead.

At that point respectability beckoned in the form of Jean Aberbach, who was one of the most powerful music publishers in America. His mother decided that I might make him a suitable wife and he decided to give me a job at Hill and Range as his firm's in-house legal counsel. I was under-qualified and overwhelmed. When Aberbach told me he wanted me to act as hostess at the firm's Christmas party, I became frightened.

It was at this point that Richard called from London, during the middle of a board meeting, and asked me how I would like to marry him. I think I said something like 'My reactions are affirmative', but afterwards left the meeting, called him back and explained I was only joking. 'OK,' said Richard, 'at least come and spend Christmas with me in England.' Aberbach announced that he would fire me if I went and that was the decisive factor in my going. Meanwhile, my mother, who desperately yearned for me to settle down, was taken with Richard and considered him an ideal candidate, unusual enough to marry her daughter.

Richard courted her by telephone as well as me, and sent flowers to us both. He wrote my father a long erudite letter asking for my hand, which sent both my parents running for the dictionary and calling upon my sister Diana to translate the English to them. When I told her about Richard's invitation, she said simply, 'Go'.

My mother came to love Richard Weston as a son. He was the only one who could persuade her to sit down at table instead of serving us all the time. He was the only one from whom she could accept a gift with obvious pleasure; the only one who could tease her. I felt this was a special relationship — in a sense my gift to her to express my gratitude for her loving me so completely that the world became a place in which I could only succeed and live happily ever after.

She began buying for me what amounted almost to a trousseau, and my girlfriend Barbara suggested to me that losing a few pounds wouldn't hurt. The current craze was for Metrecal, so she and I went to the Bronx and bought a six months' supply at reduced rates.

Losing weight made the hated shopping trips less onerous and for the first time I began to enjoy buying clothes. Before the diet I would have been a hefty size 16 or 18 — now everything started looking lots better in a size 14.

Richard's parents always spent Christmas at a luxury hotel in Torquay, so when I arrived in England we drove down to join them. I was stunned by it all, it was so very traditionally English. Everyone was extremely well dressed, well spoken, charming and interesting. It was holiday time and the food was lavish. It was like Thanksgiving with a capital T back home. I tasted Christmas Pudding for the first time and fell in love with English minted peas and, of course, Yorkshire Pudding.

What is more the sweet trolley was unbelievable. We didn't have sweet trolleys in America but at the Excelsior Hotel it was brought around during both lunch and dinner. I enjoyed it so much that Richard even arranged for them to produce it for us at breakfast.

Later I came to realize that Richard and his mother shared an obsession with food. At English restaurants in New York the portions served were notoriously meagre by American standards. I was delighted, nay, thrilled that the Westons were as enthusiastic about food as was the Turkewitz clan. Richard's mother was notorious for reaching over and putting yet another slice of meat or an extra potato on your plate when the waiter came round. Like Richard she adored gourmet food and frequently visited the most famous restaurants. They would vie for the honour of who ate what and where and cooked by whom; it was part of their normal conversation. Consequently Lillian and Bob Weston would gain weight and frequently go on diets together. Fortunately for me Richard's mother was convinced that everything new and modern came from America, particularly the latest and best diets, and thus I became a celebrity in her eyes and felt less self-conscious about my weight.

On Boxing Day, which was also my birthday, Richard asked me to marry him. To this day, I am really not certain why I agreed. Yes, it was an impetuous thing to do; we were both impetuous. Richard was bright, funny and more attentive than anyone I had ever known. His desire for me gave me a feeling of security and a greater sense of my own worth. Before, everyone I had known who was dashing and attractive wanted to redo me — slim me down and make me over. The thrill about being with Richard was that he didn't want to do that. He found me attractive the way I was.

Richard was not prepared to leave things at an engagement. He knew intuitively that if I returned home to my family, my friends, my work, my political aspirations, and thought carefully about the changes marriage to an Englishman would bring, I might well change my mind.

He began to construct our marriage service around my sense of fantasy. I had always dreamed of being married by a ship's captain. He discovered that the *Flandred*, a French ship, was completing a cruise and returning to Le Havre, with a brief stop at Southampton. He was determined that I should not return to America before we had actually been married and within one week he arranged everything. He had me dressed in a white suit and matching hat (which my mother had purchased as a 'knockout' present for me before I left for England). Soon I found myself in a small launch being taken out to the liner, while Richard convinced the two other passengers aboard — who were diplomats —to act as the witnesses in our shipboard marriage.

It all happened so fast, seemed so romantic, that I hardly took it seriously. But at midnight of January 5—6th 1963, after the marriage service, we stood on the deck of the ship alone and pledged ourselves to one another under the stars. That made it seem sacred and I took *that* pledge seriously.

We had a brief but hilarious 'half-honeymoon'. I didn't really consider that ours was a true marriage, although the captain recorded it in the ship's log, since there was no canopy and no rabbi to confirm our marriage.

I then flew back to New York to close down my office and prepare for our 'real' wedding. Even then I really wasn't consciously in love with Richard. But his daily letters, his phone calls, his poetry, his constancy and romance — and perhaps, more important, my concentrated attention on him — made me yearn for him and miss him terribly. Suddenly I knew I loved him.

A month before our religious service, Richard made an unexpected trip to New York from India. I knew as soon as I saw him that I wanted him all to myself. Although most of my family had not as yet met him and were anxious to do so, I took him straight off from the airport and drove four hours to Montauk Point on Long Island — a deserted winter resort, but beautiful at that time of year — and with no hesitation we consummated our marriage. My commitment to him was new, total and complete.

The religious ceremony duly took place in March and was a joyous Jewish celebration. We honeymooned in Mexico and by April we had set up home in England. It was a magic carpet ride — but the magic soon wore off.

I was desperately unhappy in England. Richard had found a flat for us while I was still in America and worked hard to prepare it for his new bride. It was a beautiful flat, overlooking the river in Kingston-upon-Thames (or Kingston-up-the-Thames as my mother and American friends used to call it). It had been decorated and furnished by the previous owner and was almost complete, but the main drawback was that it was out of London and I felt isolated, far from the cultural life I had known and cut off from people with whom I had rapport. Most of the other apartment owners were older, retired people and although I tried to busy myself with wifely duties, I did not have enough to do. I was plagued by fatigue and nausea, bored, lonely and frightened by what I considered to be my ill health.

The principal problem was that Richard and I didn't know or understand each other. Sure it was romantic and impetuous to get married after so short a time, but being an American, I thought all English people were automatically well educated and cultured if they spoke as well as Richard did. As a lawyer myself, I assumed he was university-educated and was astonished to discover he had little interest in books, music, politics, art or philosophy. His training at Pritchard Englefield in the technical aspects of being a solicitor was excellent; to this he added a quickness and charm which endeared him to both partners and clients. He was brilliant, highly intelligent, inventive, a master showman; yet in London I began to realise what else Richard was — or rather wasn't.

Richard was not only economical with the truth, he was extremely frugal with it. Religion soon raised problems between us. I came from a Jewish, charitable, Zionist, very politically committed home, and on his father's side Richard did too. He revered his paternal grandparents, but unfortunately, after his father's death, a quarrel between his mother and his grandparents severed all contact between the two branches of the family. After our marriage he transferred the affection he had had for his grandparents to my parents and, particularly, to my mother. So it was a shock to discover in England that Richard had mixed views about his Jewishness. It was hurtful and disturbing to encounter his family's attitudes towards educated women, contributions to charity, dedication to political or religious involvement. Moreover, I found I had married into a family where there was no discussion of art or literature — no discussion of anything but material possessions, luxury holidays, jewellery, cars, and food.

As a lawyer I enjoyed talking shop with my friends. Richard would leave the office at five and come home wanting only to enjoy his dinner and his wife.

Richard's interests were food, motor racing, boats, rugby, and me. One of the first things he did when we moved into the flat (apart from moving the furniture to show me how cricket was played) was to initiate me into the arts of making Yorkshire Pudding and all his favourite dressings and sauces. He loved meat. When he took me to Simpson's in the Strand he would tip the carver so he kept coming back offering more. He used to cut up his food with all the finesse and skill of a surgeon. His idea of pudding in a restaurant was to have them bring the trolley and then choose a helping of everything — profiteroles, chocolate mousse, trifle, crème caramel — piled on to one or two plates.

My need for fine music was frequently dismissed by a 'Could you turn that down please?' Even visits to the cinema were dictated by which theatre was closest to his favourite restaurant. He was impossibly food-orientated. As Jean Nidetch — who founded Weight Watchers in America — once remarked, 'Richard Weston's love affair with food is the purest love I have ever encountered.'

It wasn't a matter of right or wrong, or whose attitudes were more correct: it merely became painfully clear that we had little in common. I did share his lively interest in food. Both of us also had a love of stories, unusual people and outlandish situations. Our fund of jokes and anecdotes was endless; frequently we did a double act, entertaining naturally at dinner parties and other gatherings. We complemented each other, in this way, and enjoyed each other's storytelling gifts. We were a popular couple who shared a special magic at certain moments of our lives.

We were both very athletic, talented in sports and afraid of nothing. There was a powerful physical attraction between us: he loved me and I certainly loved him. I don't think I ever stopped loving Richard Weston. But I was deeply unhappy. I found myself alone most of the day with little to do as Richard had engaged a daily for the housework and I was also feeling sick most of the time. I would prepare dinner for Richard, as any young bride would do, but by the time he came home I couldn't even sit in the room with him while he ate, I was just so nauseous. It seems amusing now that neither of us suspected the reason.

I became more and more desperate and, after a row, took my car and ran away. But where to run? To an American girl (an English major) it had to be Shakespeare country. After a day or so there I moved on to Oxford, checked into the Randolph Hotel and promptly went off to a Chinese restaurant. Feeling sick hadn't made me stop thinking about food or feeling hungry. In my head I was hungry all the time. The idea of Chinese food was reassuring: it reminded me of home in America. Jewish people in New York frequented Chinese restaurants so much that we joked that if a rabbi wanted to make an important announcement, he wouldn't make it in a synagogue: he'd make it in the Chinese restaurants in Brooklyn.

As I sat there, feeling very alone and miserable, a woman in a mink coat walked in and I realised she looked terribly familiar. She looked at me as she passed my table and I realized it was Barbra Streisand with her new husband, the actor Elliott Gould. Barbra and I had met in New York during a legal case. She recognized me and asked me to join them for dinner.

As we talked I told her how unhappy I'd been and she was very sympathetic. We walked back to the Randolph where we were all staying, but just as we arrived I felt dreadfully sick. I asked her to hold my coat and raced off to the ladies' cloakroom.

On my return she wanted to know what was the matter. I explained and she immediately asked if I had considered the possibility that I was pregnant. I hadn't. I was absolutely stunned and didn't know what to do except to see a doctor.

Shamefacedly I rang Richard and asked him to arrange it. I insisted on seeing the specialist alone, for I had already decided that if his diagnosis proved negative I was going back home to America for good. However, the doctor confirmed Streisand's diagnosis and I was left with a double decision to make — about what I wanted to do with my life and the life I was carrying.

After I'd seen the doctor in London, I arranged to meet Richard and told him the news. He was overjoyed and his joy was contagious. The combination of the news and seeing Richard again, even after a short absence, made me realize how much we wanted and needed each other. The feeling of having created something together, something we could build on, something which would bind us together, overcame all fear and uncertainty.

It was a dreadful pregnancy. I couldn't keep any food down and became thinner than I'd ever been since the age of 11. In the past my weight had shifted several times a year between 10½ stone (approximately 67 kilos) to as much as 14 (approximately 89 kilos). By slimming down for my wedding I had reached a respectable size 14, but now I weighed just over 7½ stone (48 kilos). Richard didn't lose weight — in fact, because we were having all these struggles in our marriage, he resorted more and more to food.

He was a classic night eater. Because I was my mother's daughter I used to buy much too much food — I used to worry about there being a shortage in the house or that something that someone wanted at midnight might not be there — so I would buy a massive joint and cook it for dinner on Saturday night.

I reasoned that we could always use up the leftovers in sandwiches or have cold beef on Sunday, but somehow it rarely happened that way. On a Sunday morning I would come down to find the interior of the fridge looking as if a bomb had exploded — every ounce of the eight-pound joint gone! So were the biscuits. And the candy. And the ice cream — all were gone, consumed by Richard. It was a beginning without an end.

At this stage neither food nor eating habits were an issue between us. There were other issues however that proved divisive. The pregnancy did not bring us closer together for long, and I felt increasingly homesick. Richard arranged for me to go back to New York for a while and there, for the first time, I began to realize how attractive I could be if I was thin. For the first time I began to see myself as an attractive woman in my own eyes, not just in Richard's.

Our first child, Douglas, was born in England in January, 1964. Even in the hospital, amazed and delighted though we were by our new son, Richard and I quarrelled over whether or not the baby should be circumcized as part of a religious ceremony. I missed my family at the time and felt lonely and confused. When I cried the nurse came in, saying it was sad that we argued because together we brought 'sunshine to everyone'.

After Douglas's birth, things did not improve between us. At first it mattered less because I was madly in love with being a mother and adored our son. He was a constant source of delight and astonishment and I found much to keep me busy. He was the playmate I yearned for and I took him with me everywhere, even to museums, art galleries, afternoon concerts and sightseeing.

Richard became jealous of this new love affair; I suppose I made him feel left out. He decided we were going skiing, quickly found a nanny to remain at home with the baby, booked the most expensive hotel in Switzerland and announced we were going on a two-week holiday. He began a starvation diet and indeed lost weight rapidly enough to fit into tight-fitting racing stretch pants. I thought he looked marvellous.

The food in the hotel was our undoing; Richard regained all he had lost within days, and I also 'bloomed'. On top of this expensive stay, Richard decided impetuously that we should accompany another couple for a short stay at the Palace Hotel in St Moritz, reputedly one of the most expensive hotels in the world.

When we returned, my joy at being back with my baby was diminished by Richard's confession that he had blown all of his liquid assets, cashed in our wedding gift bonds, and that our joint account was in overdraft. It became clear that I had to go back to work. I couldn't bear leaving the baby and for the first time in my life wanted to stay at home. I luckily found work for American law firms who needed research papers which I could do at home, copyright lawyers then being in short supply in England, but I couldn't earn enough that way, so soon found a job with a talent agency in London.

This was exciting and challenging but Richard disapproved, because he didn't trust 'theatre people'. We began to quarrel and things became unbearable for us both. I moved out because Richard wouldn't, and began living in different flats loaned by concerned friends until I became exhausted and the baby became fretful, trying to adjust to the constant changes. I decided to leave everything, took Douglas and flew home to New York.

It was wonderful being back in Brooklyn; my family and friends made me feel cherished and valuable. Everyone spoilt, loved and admired Douglas. I intended not to return to England.

But Richard began a second course of wooing and arrived in New York, this time anxious to talk. My mother suggested that we consult a marriage counsellor who might make it easier for us to communicate.

Dr Franzblau felt that our mutual attraction was overpowering. He believed that this power could enable Richard to learn to communicate and share. He counselled Richard to change his habits of secretiveness and instability, and suggested we move from remote Kingston to a place where I would not feel so isolated. I should not make Richard feel so left out because of my attention to the baby.

We found a charming house in Datchet, Buckinghamshire, a mile from Windsor. It was a community with many other young mothers, and many intelligent and artistic people. Soon I was pregnant again. This pregnancy was not unlike the first but I also developed problems with varicose veins in my legs, trying to cope with a toddler while decorating and redoing a new house. I began to seek comfort in food once again, and because I was advised to 'put my feet up' whenever possible, I soon became fatter and fatter.

Richard used to come home with a varied assortment of meals from Harrods or Selfridges(he never trusted the local butchers) and the kosher food I loved — things like knishes, latkes and salt beef. During the day I ate biscuits, and I discovered Cadbury's chocolate and Mars bars which I used to buy twelve at a time, eat three and put the rest in the freezer to eat as a frozen dessert later.

Graeme was born in 1966. Like Douglas, he was a big baby and so very beautiful. I dreamed of coming home to burn my maternity clothes but found like so many other young mothers before me that those were the only clothes that would fit.

With two children and a new home needing improvements, Richard found a solicitor's salary inadequate for our needs. We decided together to chance a promising but highly speculative import and export trading venture. It required that we invest all our assets and commit ourselves further by borrowing heavily. We risked and we lost. The other partners weathered the storm but we were now living on twenty pounds per week with a huge mortgage and no prospects. But we had entered the project together. We were young, bright and resourceful. I am proud to say there were no quarrels over this.

Then my sister's youngest child, our beloved Hilary, died of leukaemia, having been seriously ill for the past two years. I borrowed money for my air fare and left immediately for the funeral. Richard assured me that he would find a way to bring the children and join me as soon as possible.

My parents were devastated by Hilary's death and witnessing the pain of my sister and her husband. My mother in particular was exhausted from her constant rounds of 'helping' and sharing my sister's burden and grief.

Richard arrived with the boys and suggested we take my parents away to Florida where my brother lived. He wisely suggested that seeing their grandsons after a long absence would distract my parents and give my mother a new focus. We lied about our financial condition, explaining that the British had imposed a fifty-pound travel allowance 'quota' and we were limited in terms of funds we could remove from England.

My parents were delighted to treat us as their guests and my mother chose a small, inexpensive, unimpressive motel where she could do all the cooking in what my sons called 'Bubby's restaurant'. Richard loved my mother and her cooking — but hated poverty more. He cringed at the aged car we had to rent and sought comfort, as always, in food.

We were both outsize by this time; having finished a diet shortly before we left England, we succumbed to the lure of Miami delicatessens. We regained everything we had lost as well as adding, in my case, half a stone and in Richard's, a stone and a half. My brother, a heart specialist, was appalled at our yo-yo syndrome of gaining, losing and regaining, and cautioned us against it. He advised us to deal with our obesity more sensibly and suggested that we try a new group therapy approach which had recently been launched in Miami. It was called Weight Watchers. Several of Hy's patients who were seriously ill had been greatly helped by losing weight and maintaining their loss sensibly with Weight Watchers. He gave us a copy of the diet early one morning and we went off to Wolfie's famous restaurant to have breakfast and read it. Our waitress was the most emaciated woman in the world, or so it seemed to me. She noticed that Richard had the Weight Watchers diet sheet in his hand — and she immediately removed the wholemilk and the sugar from the table, replacing them with sweet-ener and another kind of milk which looked very thin.

Richard started ordering; he wanted four eggs well done, hot buttered toast, bacon not too crisp with grilled toma-toes, and a side-order of griddle cakes. The waitress listened but wrote nothing down.

When Richard completed his order, she said: 'Uh, uh — you can't have anything like that. Isn't that a Weight Watchers diet you've got there?'

Richard was annoyed, but I was intrigued. How could this skinny thing know about diets, and why did she care what he ate? I asked her what he 'could' have and she recited verbatim a perfect Weight Watchers breakfast, lunch and dinner menu. She explained that her boss obliged the staff to memorize the entire Weight Watchers programme; she even brought us a specially printed Weight Watchers menu and that truly impressed me. If a restaurant famous for its rich food would go to these lengths, they must have considered it good for business.

The waitress confirmed that it was. Women on diets usually avoided restaurants — the temptation was too great. When they stayed away, so did their husbands and children. By making it possible for dieters to eat Weight Watchers style, the whole family continued to patronize the restaurant and everyone benefitted. Now I was even more interested and so was Richard — interested enough to resolve to go to a Weight Watchers class that very night. For the rest of the day we ate as if every meal was our last. We ordered three portions of Wolfie's Victory Cake which consisted of eight layers of pure whipped cream with chocolate interspersed; it was called 'Victory' because few people ever managed to complete the portion served. Richard kept me talking. I was quite verbose and he managed to eat his portion and the third before I was aware of what he was doing.

We had a big lunch with my mother and the children, then we went and ate again. We said we were going out shopping, but we went to Pumperniks, a marvellous place like Wolfie's only better because it made its own black bread. We ate all the bread and pickles on the table, then we had chicken soup with noodles. Richard had a plate of hot pastrami with more pickles. We each had a frankfurter and for dessert Richard had more soup. But we did buy a case of diet Tab and another of diet Pepsi to take back to the hotel. We kidded ourselves that if we drank slimming drinks our sins would float away.

Of course, what we were doing was preparing to be in jail for the rest of our lives, because that's just how you feel when you are about to go on a diet. We had no idea how different it would be with Weight Watchers.

Weight Watchers was started in America by Jean Nidetch, who had been fat ever since childhood. She used to say that she believed that when she was a child in her pram a wicked fairy had put a curse on her: that she would always have a beautiful face, always be fat, and always be intelligent enough to be hurt by it.

Having been on every conceivable diet, she was in a supermarket one day when she ran into a friend who told her she looked marvellous and enquired when the baby was due. Since Jean wasn't pregnant, she was very upset, so when she heard about a programme being run at the New York City Board of Health obesity clinic, she joined.

She went along to her first session and found it was being run by a very thin nurse. Her opening line was to ask the class how they would react after eating their fill if they were tempted by a new offer of delicious food. Before anyone could answer, the nurse added, 'I would be sick to my stomach.'

At this point Jean realized there was an unbridgeable gap between them. How could anyone feel sick looking at food? she wondered. How could anyone who had never been fat understand fat people and the way they behave?

However, Jean attended regularly for ten weeks, gave up ice cream, and pizza and cake, ate the prescribed meals — and lost an average two pounds per week. It would have been more but for the fact that she just could not resist eating biscuits — and she could not admit to a teacher so lacking in sympathy and understanding that she had been cheating.

In the end, Jean took the programme (which was originally written by Dr Norman Joliffe) and persuaded some of her overweight friends to follow it with her, for moral support. They decided to meet every week in her house, to talk, swap stories and help each other stick to the diet. After two weeks Jean realised she was getting more from these meetings than she was from the clinic, and never went back. The group chipped in and bought a pair of medical scales and started to keep a record of the weekly weigh-in.

Gradually word spread and more and more women came until there were so many they had to meet in the basement of Jean's apartment block. At first Jean didn't charge. If people couldn't get to her — because they were too fat to get behind the wheel of a car, or they just never went out — she went to them. If someone called up and said they were in the Bronx she would find out where the Bronx was and go.

One day a woman rang to ask if she would go and talk to a group of people in Long Island and that was how she met Al and Felice Lippert. Al was a very successful salesman in the fashion industry and he and his wife were both overweight. By now Jean had instituted a system of handing out pins as rewards for losing a certain amount of weight. When she presented this group with their pins, Al Lippert told her she was acting unwisely. He advised that instead of Jean giving expensive gifts to these people, they should be buying her something as a thank you, or paying her for her services. In fact, he said, it was time for her to get truly organized and start to run a commercial business.

He gave her the money to rent a room and form a

company. Together they set up a business. On May 15th
1963 Weight Watchers was born. It just grew and grew and
grew some more. So many people wanted Weight Watchers
classes in other parts of the country that soon a franchise
system was developed. In 1966, when Richard and I encountered Weight Watchers, a franchise had been newly
opened in Miami.

I'll never forget our first encounter with Norma Frasher,
one of the two franchisees in charge of the Miami operation.
Richard and I actually arrived at the Weight Watchers office
clutching hamburgers dripping with ketchup and relish
and drinking triple thick milk shakes with extra ice cream.
Norma Frasher took one look at us and said, 'Who sent you
here — the Gestapo?'

Norma was larger than life in every respect. She was like
a stand-up comic, warm and intelligent, and she loved
being attractive and a star. She explained about Weight
Watchers, showed us her 'before' picture — her weight loss
was very impressive — and waived the usual $10 fee which
pleased Richard, I suspect, because he was trying to
convince himself that he was attending in some kind of
professional capacity and wasn't one of the dull, fat people
he expected to see.

In fact, when we arrived at the meeting we found the
people and the atmosphere far from dull. It was lively,
amusing, and very moving. The person I sat next to resem-
bled a young Cary Grant. He was absolutely beautiful and
looked as if he had never been a pound overweight. When I
asked him what he was doing there he said he had come for
his monthly 'fix'. He explained that he had lost over 100
pounds a year and a half ago, and came to class each month
as part of his free lifetime membership. What knocked me
sideways was not that he had lost all that weight — I could
lose weight — but the fact that he had maintained that
weight loss for such a long time. No one I knew had ever
maintained a weight loss for a month, let alone a year and a
half, and no one I knew who had been on a serious diet had

ever looked that well and so naturally slim after such a large weight loss.

I was impressed by the eating programme as well: it stressed that you were cheating if you did not eat everything you were supposed to and it allowed you to eat between meals. I couldn't have done without my 'snacks'. What Weight Watchers offered instead was a sensible list of 'free' foods which were crunchy and tasty and which you could nibble on at any time.

We both began losing weight, to our delight, and neither of us felt hungry. This was the first time Richard had been on a diet which he did not associate with starvation, and by the time he had to return to England, he had already lost almost a stone. He soon rang me from Datchet and said, 'Listen, if you don't bring Weight Watchers over here, and we don't continue going to meetings, we will both get fat again.'

He was right, but he had also seen the business possibilities. He had counted the number of people who turned up each week at our class and at other classes we visited just for fun. He concluded that Weight Watchers had great financial promise and might be a way out of our immediate money difficulties. He saw it only as a short-term solution whereby we could augment his income, pay off some immediate debts and have a little money to live on. In his eyes it was something we could do for a year or so, not a business venture which would make our fortune.

Richard was a risk-taker and thought we had nothing to lose. He would only have accepted it on a short-term basis because running Weight Watchers was not dignified enough for him. He was even reluctant to tell our neighbours and his colleagues about our plans. I think he seriously didn't believe Weight Watchers could work well or for long in the United Kingdom. It was a therapy-oriented approach that would not appeal to the reticent British. I wasn't thinking in those terms at all. I was unhappy and felt unfulfilled in England. Suddenly there was a wonderful opportunity to start something that was interesting, worth-while, challenging and fun. It might help us solve our weight problems, and was a concept that I truly respected and believed in.

When we first inquired about obtaining a franchise, the Americans were amused. To them England was a place in history — somewhere far across the ocean. I was impressed with their sincerity, however, and their conviction that only fat people who had lost weight with Weight Watchers were truly eligible to be franchisees and would bring to the business the care, concern and understanding that members need. They said that in order to qualify I must train as a lecturer and visit as many classes as possible. I went to many different locations, observing as many classes as possible. I visited an average of three or four a day and found each class and every lecturer more interesting than the last.

Although all followed the same rules and regulations, each was different and all were extremely entertaining. At a class in Queens, New York, I heard the real definition of a seafood diet — it's one where you eat everything you see.

Then there was Sophie who ran a class in Flatbush, near my mother's home. More than a hundred people would pack the room just to hear her, she was so amusing. She told us the story of the time when she tried to marry off her daughter.

'I was a big fat thing,' she said, 'with a daughter who was reasonably sized. We figured that any boy who came into the house would have been told by his mother, "Take a look at the mother to see what the daughter will look like after twenty years." So I knew I had to do something. I joined Weight Watchers and lost weight and so did my daughter.

'Then suddenly she attracted a very nice boy. She announced that he was coming to call on her — so we organized everything nicely and I stayed home to meet him. What I forgot was I have a big-mouth son. While this boy was sitting in the living room waiting to court my daughter, my son introduced himself and said, "You should have seen my sister before, the fat slob, and you should have seen my mother!" Then he started taking out the photo albums. Well, I came as close as ever I hope to be to committing murder in my own house. But that,' she said, 'is one of the things you have to contend with.'

I learned a tremendous amount from Sophie and from the other lecturers. Some scolded members who had cheated, some used the 'you-can't-let-me-down' technique, but the best value by far came from the entertainers who hypnotized their audiences with their exuberance and joy. Each class was different, depending on the personality of the lecturer and of the members who completed the group. It was this difference of approach that inspired me, like variations on a theme in music, to believe that I, too, could create my own melody which the British would learn to sing, or even just to hum.

I can't honestly say that Richard and I had any deep discussions about whether or not we should go ahead. (Before Weight Watchers Richard and I never really had deep discussions about anything.) In a sense we were simply carried along on a wave of enthusiasm. My mother thought it was a good idea, and the American Weight Watchers thought we were cute kids and were keen for us to go ahead. They wanted $2,500 for the English franchise, plus a royalty of ten per cent of our gross income. Since we had no money at all that seemed a great deal to pay up front. In hindsight, it was a wise move on their part to make us pay the franchise fee before we even started. It was an incentive for us to make it work.

We borrowed the money from my mother. Even she didn't see it as a form of investment. She saw it as a gift.

CHAPTER THREE

I had reached goal weight in New York, finalized the franchise agreement and returned to England ready to open our first Weight Watchers centre. I found that Richard had regained some weight because he no longer had any class to attend. I believed that if this was to be our business, if we were to inspire and direct others, we ourselves should be role models and follow the Programme scrupulously. Richard agreed and together we gave away all the sugar, oil, butter, peanuts, crisps and Mars bars we had in the house.

But it involved much greater sacrifices than that because Richard was a great meat eater and found it difficult to limit his meat eating to three times a week, and I never thought I could eat five fish meals a week. I simply hated fish.

Soon, however, we found that eating Weight Watchers style full-time became a habit which was acceptable to us and actually enjoyable. We cooked together, inventing recipes and acceptable substitutes, and came to love Weight Watchers soups, milk shakes, salad dressings and sauces.

It meant we could eat puddings so we experimented, creating wonderful desserts such as cherry cheesecake and apple and blackberry mousse: we soon discovered it was easier to eat in restaurants, too, and we didn't have to curtail our social life. Although I was permitted to follow a maintenance regime and have extras, out of loyalty to Richard I stuck to the basic diet and continued to lose weight, going half a stone below goal. Richard never reached goal which was a serious mistake because one needs that special magic of setting a target and attaining it.

Still, he lost four stone and looked youthful and handsome.

We both had always been energetic, annoyingly so to many who knew us. Now we had inexhaustible energy, all of which we channelled into founding, developing and directing Weight Watchers UK.

Richard took full charge of setting up the company and handled the financial, legal and administrative aspects. It was a Weight Watchers joke for many years that Bernice Weston's weekly tally sheet was simply called 'the sheet' because it never tallied. It would annoy Richard, who was meticulous, to find my shopping lists and personal reminders on the back of the tally sheet. But I was working as a housewife, running an office at home with no nanny, no secretary, no nothing; I had to improvise while we created a business.

Later it was to be a source of great irritation to Richard, and a great comfort to me, that many of the women who worked with us committed the same clerical crimes. Richard was forced to create special systems for them, frequently calling upon their husbands to help straighten out the paperwork.

Because Richard was away all day at the office, I was left to find a location for our first class. We originally planned to open in Golders Green, in north London: it was the nearest equivalent we could think of to Brooklyn, where Weight Watchers had been so successful. When we visited classes in Brooklyn we were given the names of English relatives of some American Weight Watchers who assured us that Golders Green was just waiting for us to start.

Meanwhile at the Datchet keep-fit class run by Eileen Fowler, I was introduced to a neighbour, Barbara Hardwick. She told me that she needed an operation on her leg, but that doctors were delaying surgery until she reduced her weight. 'You must help me,' she said. 'I can't get to Golders Green, it's too far. If you open in Datchet, I'll join and help you.' Despite Richard's objections that he didn't want us to run a class in our own village, I finally convinced him that it would be easier for me to run the class and the office, while still minding the children, if I did not have to travel too far.

We began with a free open meeting which we advertized locally. Sixteen people attended: some were personal friends; some had heard about Weight Watchers through the leaflets we had asked the local Boy Scouts to distribute; others were just curious. Barbara Hardwick didn't show up at all. When Richard wanted to know where she was, I convinced him that she was already sold on the idea and would be at the first official meeting. In fact she didn't join for some time — until her best friend lost weight and became slimmer than she.

Richard and I really had no idea how much to say or how long to talk: we were nervous but so enthusiastic that we talked solidly for two and a half hours. It was like a vaudeville show and everyone laughed. Then I wrapped it up, explaining how Weight Watchers worked, and how they could join.

We held the first official meeting the following week, March 3rd, 1967. We charged £1 to register and 14 shillings (70 pence) for each weekly meeting. This time, only three people showed up.

Maureen Toulson was Britain's first Weight Watchers member. At 32, she weighed 11 st 7 lb (approximately 73 kilos) but seven months later she had slimmed down to a trim 8 st 6 lb (55 kilos). As a friend she shared our enthusiasm, following the diet even before classes officially began. She held the first membership card, was the first to reach goal, the first lecturer to train and open her own class in St Albans. In the midst of all crises she always saw the funny side and her laughter would ring out infectiously and calm everyone. Nutritional scientists were fascinated by the length of her successful weightloss maintenance and as a registered nurse she became our skilled spokeswoman to the medical profession. Once, when she was racing to a training session at my home with a bumper sticker on her car saying 'Help Stamp Out Obesity — Follow Me to Weight Watchers', she was stopped by a policeman. He said that he would help her stamp out obesity if she would help him stamp out speeding!

Maureen brought her mother, Alice Noble, to that first meeting. She was an active, well-spoken club woman whose husband was an executive in the City. At the other end of the social spectrum was our third member, Irene Belcher, the actor Donald Pleasance's daily.

All three came back the second week and as I weighed Irene we discovered she had lost 4 pounds. She was so delighted that she jumped off the scales and slapped Mrs Noble on the back from sheer joy, exclaiming, 'I lost four pounds in a week, ducky!' Seeing this interaction between the daily and the executive wife, Richard turned to me and whispered, 'You have just seen the demise of Weight Watchers in Great Britain.' How wrong he was. When Mrs Noble discovered she had lost the same amount as Irene, they joined arms and did a kind of jig around the hall. It just proved that not only were fat women sisters under the skin, but that Weight Watchers was classless.

The early days were both difficult and great fun. Mrs Noble brought along her neighbour, a lovely woman called Joyce Gourdie. She had been a hospital sister who was married late in life to an extremely successful company secretary. She was in her sixties and had been advised to lose weight because she had a bad heart. Joyce was softly spoken, understated, but always beautifully turned out. Once, when I was in distress, with no babysitter and a class to run, she offered to help by staying with my children. When I returned she was in total disarray but happy, and she volunteered again and again. She even did my washing up. Later, when we were invited to have tea with her, I met the large staff in her impressive house and she confessed that she hadn't washed a dish at home in years.

When, at a later date, I prohibited all our lecturers, clerks and weighers from wearing trousers, I was amused to see her husband Ronnie, a Scot, arrive at one of our social occasions dressed in a kilt. When I told him how original I thought his costume was, he said, 'No costume, ma'am. I'm Joyce's clerk and you have forbidden me to wear trousers.'

Joyce brought along another new member, and that's how it went. Someone would come, and someone would leave. No matter what we did, we never seemed to hold more than six or eight members in the class and that continued until the local paper publicized the successes of our members after our first sixteen-week award-giving ceremony.

Among our earliest members were three women from Gerrards Cross who went on to become very important in Weight Watchers. Betty Clark was a compulsive eater who put on weight easily and took it off slowly. When she joined she was 12st 9lb (82 kilos), but through Weight Watchers she learned to control her eating and went on to run our workshop training centres. Betty had a rare gift: the ability to teach. She trained ordinary people to understand the basics of nutrition, to answer Weight Watchers' questions, to speak from their own experience, to be confident, efficient and inspiring without imitating others: not easy things to do.

June Leonard had been the proverbial professional dieter and she joined Weight Watchers purely because it was yet another new thing to try. When she walked through the doors of the Datchet class in March she was 40 and weighed 14st 13lb (90 kilos) — but by September she had reached her goal weight of 9st 10lb (63 kilos), shedding 4st 3lb (27 kilos) on the way.

Pat Gregory also lost weight quickly and became one of our most joyful publicists. She went everywhere, telling anyone who would listen how she had slimmed down from 12st 12lb (81 kilos) to 9st 13lb (64 kilos) in just sixteen weeks. But not all Pat's friends were as pleased about her new slim figure as she was. In fact, the very friend who had told her about Weight Watchers suddenly started bringing her chocolates — a not so subtle form of sabotage. It emerged that the 'friend' resented losing Pat as a free baby-sitter. Now that Pat's social life had blossomed and her figure improved, she became a much sought after dinner guest speaker and we soon sent her around the county, speaking to women's groups about Weight Watchers.

One of the secrets of the success of Weight Watchers was that the classes were structured so that issues like 'sabotage' could be aired. People came along, paid their weekly fee, stood on the scales and had their weight recorded. Then the lecturer welcomed the group, introduced herself, and presented a carefully structured theme which stimulated group discussion, before calling on everybody in turn to tell their stories and join in with their opinions as she read out their weight losses. She invited each one to share an important feeling, to relate an experience or to ask a question. It was during these discussion times that all kinds of problems were raised.

Doubters warned us that anything which smacked of group therapy would simply not work in England. In fact, one of the marvellous things about our classes was the way in which people did 'open up'. They knew they were in the company of others who had faced the same pain and problems; they cheered the successful and encouraged the unsuccessful. It was a wonderful place to make new friends. Fat people had fewer social opportunities and, for some, this class was the high point of their week.

From the very beginning I felt honoured to work with such lovely and interesting women (and the few men who bravely joined). As they responded to me and opened up to each other, I felt a sense of pride and satisfaction at being accepted as one of them.

Very early on it became clear that although the structure of the weekly meetings had crossed the Atlantic without any trouble, the same could not be said for the dietary programme itself. It was very difficult to find low-calorie drinks and almost impossible to obtain skimmed milk (one of the staples of our diet) except in huge catering packs.

I rang Al Lippert in New York, as one Brooklynite to another, and asked for his help. I told him that an American Rothschild had volunteered to bring us a large supply of powdered skimmed milk from America but only if it was delivered direct to her stateroom on a transatlantic liner. Not only did Al promise to help but he delivered all the cartons himself. She promptly tipped him! We roared with laughter for years afterwards at that story.

The American diet sheet referred to certain New York specialities such as bagels and gefilte fish, and certain fruits and vegetables were confusingly known by different names: courgettes were called zucchini, aubergines, eggplants. Although the early members were prepared to go to great lengths to find delicatessens and other specialist shops, we soon realized we would have to anglicize the programme. With Jean Nidetch's blessing we hired our own specialist in nutrition and revised the diet. Soon we retained our own medical and psychological advisers, all of whom worked in splendid co-operation with their American counterparts.

As the summer approached we were still struggling to build the class membership at Datchet up to ten. Richard and I received a phone call from Norma Frasher in Miami Beach who wanted to know how we were getting on. 'Fine,' we bluffed. Then she went on, 'Gee, things are really quiet here — we're almost a thousand members down this week.'

After we'd put down the phone Richard and I gulped and looked at each other. We really began to wonder if we were doing it all wrong. Norma was worrying about losing a thousand members, we were worrying about getting into double figures. Would Weight Watchers ever really take off in England? Still, at the same time we were enjoying ourselves; we liked the people, we liked what we were doing, and we were learning a tremendous amount.

Most important of all, Richard and I were getting along better than ever before. We were working on something together and it gave us cause to have deep discussions and to share many experiences. We complemented each other extremely well. Richard was magnificently unself-conscious about racing to and fro, setting up the chairs, lugging the scales and hanging up the pictures. He greeted all the members warmly, gave brilliant lectures, or joined me in a comic routine to lighten the atmosphere. He dealt brilliantly with all the administrative details; perhaps more vital than anything, he encouraged me whenever I felt inadequate and unsure. He was the natural showman who taught me to find my own place in the limelight.

In the early days there were certainly times when we both needed a good dose of encouragement. Our choice of location for a second class was St John's Wood, a smart and expensive area of London. It was a dreadful mistake. Richard's mother's hairdresser had promised to bring along all her overweight clients. Two people turned up to the free open meeting (neither of them from the hairdressing salon) and none at all the following week, so we had to close the class.

At least the experience taught us not to rely on well-wishers and friends. Instead we followed our instincts: Golders Green would be next. Even this was almost a disaster.

The first free open meeting was held in a room at the Cavalier pub which we booked in advance for a four-week period. Unfortunately the publican had assumed that whatever kind of meeting we were holding would be good for his business.

When nobody ordered a drink he couldn't understand it. He later read our literature and realized that Weight Watchers banned alcohol. Without bothering to inform us he then hired out the room for the second week to someone else and when Richard — who was always early for appointments, thank goodness — arrived, the room was already occupied.

Richard raced, on foot, all the way to the Brent Bridge

Hotel, which was about half a mile away, and booked the only available room — the ballroom. That night we ferried people from the pub to the hotel in the pouring rain, knowing that the ballroom was costing us whatever we might earn in the next six months!

Later a friend suggested we use a room above the Odeon cinema at Temple Fortune, just down the road. That became one of our most successful meeting places for many years.

One of the women who joined the class in Golders Green was Rita Dijon: she was married to an American serviceman based in Ruislip. She told us there were a number of overweight Americans on the base who had been ordered to lose weight by their commanding officer. The original plan to hold a class on the base itself didn't work out, but we soon found a place nearby and service people did join, as did the local people from Northwood, Middlesex.

One was Nancy Lidell, the wife of Alvar Lidell, one of the BBC's most famous radio personalities. He became so enthusiastic about Nancy's weight loss that he memorized the entire programme, studied all her training material, and when she became a lecturer, often answered the telephone at home, giving advice to anxious members with one of the most familiar and popular voices in England. It was a hoot, and a great break for us.

At this time I became very keen on the idea of running a class in a department store. I heard it had worked well in America and the idea made sense. Women from quite a wide catchment area came up to London to do their shopping: we couldn't hope to open classes at this stage near all their homes. A class in a department store centrally located in London would attract a whole new range of members, and from the store's point of view it would be an added attraction.

With typical Brooklyn chutzpah I decided to approach Harrods first. Their reception of the proposal was one of refined disdain: 'Classes for the obese, in Harrods?' There wasn't a shred of interest, just ill-concealed amazement at our even making such a suggestion. I felt utterly dismissed, a non-person. Another lesson learned!

We then began negotiations with Gorringe's, in Victoria. While talks were going on, Richard's law partner introduced him to Rowan Bentall, owner of the famed department store in Kingston-on-Thames. Bentall's had always been my favourite store because when I was very homesick, during those early days in Kingston, I used to go down to the basement where the big American fridges used to cheer me up and make me feel more at home.

Rowan Bentall visited one of our classes with his housekeeper. He wanted her opinion on whether our diet would be manageable for a typically English housewife — and whether these were meals that would assist his own wife in watching her weight. The housekeeper was impressed and Rowan Bentall was charmed and invited us to plan for an autumn opening at his store.

By this time we had started up at Gorringe's. The members were interesting and did come from diverse backgrounds and locations. The setting was at first ideal and it was good for business at Gorringe's since we encouraged our members when they wanted to go on a binge to buy lotions and make-up instead of chocolate bars.

Later we had a row with the store because they misused the Weight Watchers name to advertize what we considered 'illegal' food. We were soon out of favour and found ourselves moved from room to room each week. At one point, as I was lecturing in a changing room, a hand reached across my face to get a dress and pulled it out right under my nose.

Because they were always moving us about, they frequently upset our scales. One week we discovered the scales were actually broken. I was now faced with a group of women who had travelled from as far away as Bromley, anxious to find out how much weight they had lost that week. I knew I could not let them leave without knowing how well they had done: even my most uplifting lecture would be no substitute for that. I suddenly had the brilliant idea of taking them into Boot's the chemist. We all trundled down the escalators in hilarious mood, and I weighed them publicly on the store's scale.

There was one occasion, though, when even Boot's couldn't come to the rescue. Pat Brown joined the class, and she was our first very, very overweight lady. She was so overweight that we couldn't weigh her on our normal medical scales. These only went up to 20 stone. Then I had the bright idea of taking her to the British Airways office nearby. Unfortunately their scales only went up to 25 stone and when the pointer swung straight past the maximum weight it was embarrassingly obvious she was even heavier than that. By this time she was pleading with me to let her go back to Bromley, but as we walked back into Victoria Station where she was going to catch her train, I spotted some huge baggage scales. I looked at them and I looked at her. 'Oh no,' she said at first. But I persuaded her to hop on while I took a quick look before anyone noticed. She weighed 26 st 10 lb (171 kilos) and went on to become one of our great successes.

Gorringe's, however, was not. We were given a week's notice and I was crestfallen. Where would I find another place for all these members in such a short time? One of the quiet women in the group disappeared during the class and then came running back, out of breath. 'We're moving to the Westminster Theatre just near here,' she announced. It turned out that the theatre was the home of the Moral Rearmament movement and she was a member. We all marched out of Gorringe's and over to the theatre that very day. Seven of us piled into the lift — and promptly broke it. The manager of the theatre was very understanding and polite. He merely said, 'I wonder if you could ask your women to use the stairs in future?'

Our eviction from Gorringe's turned out to be a blessing

in disguise. There was a dining room at the Westminster Theatre where we were able to arrange for Weight Watchers meals to be served, and it was a good place for me to invite members of the press. By coincidence Rowan Bentall was also a member of Moral Rearmament. The fact that the Westminster Theatre was happy for us to hold classes there must have helped to persuade him that we were respectable and sincere. He confirmed that we could open at Bentall's — and that was how we staged the fashion show that really put us on the map.

When you are fat the last thing you normally want to do is to go to a fashion show. It's too punishing. I had never been to one in my life and neither had most of the women in Weight Watchers. Having promised to do a fashion show I was in a panic until I read about a similar event which had taken place in America.

I decided to send out invitations to every top newspaper and magazine journalist, and then ring them, ring them, and ring again until they agreed to come. And to make sure they would come all the way to Kingston we laid on a special bus.

The models were to be Weight Watchers, some of whom had lost as much as 100 pounds (7 st 2lb, approximately 46 kilos), and who could now wear fashionable clothes for the first time in their lives. We arranged to have huge blow-ups done of their 'before' pictures and then we planned a photographic session to take some 'after' ones to use as promotional material.

The photo session was chaotic. The women turned up with dresses that were hanging shapelessly because they hadn't yet invested in new clothes. I had to rush round with pins. I even remember sitting on the floor taking up hems — I, who hardly ever sewed a stitch in my life. Later, when I showed the photos to my mother she said, 'Don't tell me who did those hems. It had to be you. You always had one hand shorter than the other when it came to sewing.'

Something significant happened at the rehearsal, too.

Rowan Bentall had agreed that we could all come in and choose what we wanted to wear. All the women immediately headed for clothes in their old size. They hadn't realized they really had lost weight, and were still afraid of trying on bright colours or anything which would draw attention to themselves. When you've been fat for a long time, old habits die hard.

But we went ahead and on September 20th 1967 the first Weight Watchers fashion show duly took place. And it wasn't just women who modelled: one lone man, our good friend Gordon Rose from the Golders Green class, was also there to show how he had slimmed down from almost 19 stone to 14 in five months. He wore the suit he joined in, then another suit underneath, and finally stripped down to a pair of modish jeans and a shirt. He brought the house down.

Everyone looked superb and the spin-off publicity value was tremendous. The journalists were welcomed with a Weight Watchers cocktail (non-alcoholic, of course) and given a seven-course Weight Watchers lunch after the show. Clement Freud wrote amusingly in the *Financial Times* about his encounter with one of our Bloody Marys (renamed a Bloody Shame).

'As Weight Watchers shun alcohol,' he observed, 'they had substituted tabasco for vodka — and tabasco you should know is a solution of cayenne and chilli pepper, served in very small drops. My cocktail contained a sizeable whoosh, as a result of which I became instantly and entirely weightless (I jumped high into the air).'

By the end of that first year we had eight classes: two in Datchet: two in Golders Green; one near Ruislip; the two which we had started at Gorringe's and transferred to the Westminster Theatre, and one in St Albans.

Richard and I were still running them all between us, although Maureen Toulson was taking the St Albans class under Richard's supervision. It was a hectic time. Up until that point the only office help I'd had was from a woman called Shirley Hillier, who used to make calls, write letters, do the ironing and babysit for me. I couldn't have managed without her but she had only taken what was meant to be a part-time job in order to brush up her skills. There was too much to do: the strain made her nervous and affected her health. Shirley used to ring Richard at his office and plead with him to get me to fire her or accept her resignation.

On the day of the fashion show I was desperate for someone to man the phone in the office at home and take care of the children. Another kind woman from one of our classes, Theresa Grosvenor, volunteered. She was very composed, very well groomed, and she told me she had never changed a nappy or done any kind of housework. By the time we got home she looked as if she had been pulled through a hedge backwards. 'This is madness,' she told me. 'How you do it every day, I'll never know.'

I wasn't sure either and it was clear some changes would have to be made. We would have to move on to a more business-like footing if Weight Watchers was to go on growing.

We moved the office from our home to a room above a turf accountant's shop at Datchet Green and advertized for an office manager. Sally Moynahan replied. She weighed 20 stone (127 kilos) — and the man working in the bookie's underneath was terrified she would come crashing through the floor one day and crush him. There were also other problems which made that office inconvenient. I called in my close friend Barbara Hardwick and soon she placated the man and devised solutions for all our problems. She even installed special sliding doors so Sally could fit into the loo.

Barbara became one of my treasures in Weight Watchers. She was a handsome heavyweight who became a striking, dramatic-looking lightweight, and was not only a valued employee but remains a cherished friend. Her poise, calm, honesty and directness commanded respect and instilled confidence and affection. Although her classes grew quickly

I seconded her as my personal assistant. Later she was appointed a director at our office in Windsor. Her knowledge of food preparation and presentation was unmatched, whilst her experience as a lecturer with her own classes made her advice invaluable: she was a perfect go-between, bringing my messages to the lecturers, supervisors and members — and vice versa. She was better than any progress reports churned out by computers and graphs.

But that lay in the future. At this stage I realized I needed to train other Weight Watchers to become lecturers, and eventually trainers and supervisors. Richard and I couldn't do it all.

This was forcibly brought home to me when Richard became ill. He had been spending so much time with Weight Watchers that he consequently spent less time at his law practice. As a result his partners asked him to choose between the two: they thought Weight Watchers diminished him and, by inference, their law practice. He didn't tell me any of this. He resigned as a partner, agreeing to remain as a consultant, then he just came home, crawled into bed and stayed there — in deep depression.

But I reacted differently. Richard retreated in hurt and confusion while I, hardy child of Brooklyn, came out fighting. I resented the implied disparagement of our work. I valued our co-workers, our group members, and our chance to help these fat sisters under the skin discover how clever, how bright, how beautiful they really were. We would show them!

If Weight Watchers were to continue to expand I realized we would have to find an administrator. We needed someone urgently — someone to plan our national growth and co-ordinate our plans for expansion.

I turned to Leslie Levonton, a former client of Richard's and a friend. Leslie and his wife Sylvia had sent us a telegram on the first night of our Datchet class which said: 'Best Wishes and Congratulations on the Birth of a New Industry.' At that time with our membership of three, it seemed a bit of a joke. But Leslie was always intrigued by the concept and prepared to back us.

I suggested that he become our Managing Director, knowing Richard would be pleased since he looked on Leslie as a pragmatic, experienced businessman to whom everyone turned in moments of need.

I was particularly drawn to Leslie because he respected women and enjoyed working with them. He was sympathetic and patient. He was the first to come to work in the morning, the last to leave at night. All details were important to him. He 'lived' Weight Watchers. Each new lecturer, new opening, new trainee, regional conference, seminar or promotional event received his careful attention. He drove hundreds of miles throughout the country each week, determined to see things for himself; he helped Richard and me weave each skein of the Weight Watchers organization into a smooth but colourful whole. He was our friend, our co-worker — and oftentimes — our referee.

Sylvia Levonton made herself available from the earliest days to help me seek out locations. She was a source of unending information and support to me, a relative stranger to the country. Sylvia became a lecturer and conducted several of our largest and most successful classes in north London. Her previous experience as an entertainer and her fashion sense were an inspiration to the younger lecturers. Her style and approach were different from mine, but her members enjoyed her engagingly strict approach. She was particularly effective with the numerous male members who profited from her no-nonsense method.

(Later, this relationship was to become strained when my determination to introduce advanced lecturing techniques and innovative psychological approaches disturbed and confused Leslie. He felt I was overloading the organization with overhead expenses which took away from our profitability. He was stubborn, as was I. We rowed. I lost a marvellous friend and Weight Watchers lost an able director. The couple who shared so many of our joys and sorrows and refereed even more of our business and domestic conflicts were sorely missed. It pleases me that their son-in-law, Barry, is still part of Weight Watchers as manager of one of their European operations.)

With Richard ill, and after a fortnight of coping with everything alone, I also knew that we had to have more lecturers. The trouble was, I didn't really know how to train them — or so I thought.

I had begun by encouraging some of the members of my Datchet class to come to sessions at my home. I would give them a theme and they would take it in turns to stand up and talk. Then we would discuss how to improve their speaking voice, their posture, their presentation, and the content of their lecture. Eight months later I was still training the initial group because I didn't know when to stop.

Luckily, at this point Fred Jaroslaw, a franchisee from New Jersey, came to England. During his stay he sat in on one of my training sessions. He was very impressed and wanted to know where the women were lecturing. When he discovered they were still training he told me I was mad. 'They're as good as anyone I've seen in America,' he said. 'Put them out to work.' So I did.

Although I over-trained this first group, that was the best mistake I ever made — because they in turn over-trained their groups, and as a result the standard of lecturers was superb and the success of Weight Watchers virtually guaranteed.

Each lecturer, when chosen to open a new class, was free to suggest a location which would be convenient for her. When that had been agreed, it was her job to find a place in which to hold the class. Then I would go along to see if it was suitable. Once it was approved I coached the lecturer as to how to approach the local newspaper with her own story and her before and after pictures. She would encourage the paper to run a story explaining that she was opening a class in the area to share the secrets of her success with future Weight Watchers members.

One of the things I learned from my experiences during my happy days as a young theatrical lawyer was the value of publicity. I didn't believe in advertizing at all; the most Weight Watchers ever did was to pay for a small ad announcing where to find local classes. Instead I worked on the theory that good journalists need good stories to write about — and I believed we had the most interesting stories. What is more, I trained my lecturers to be effective publicists: I asked them to write up what occurred in their classes each week, to include at least one anecdote or one motivating story. I encouraged them to send that report, not only to me at head office, but also to the local newspaper.

These reports were not always followed up immediately, but every now and then when a journalist or an editor was looking for a good story, these reports caught their interest and were printed — and that meant valuable free publicity for Weight Watchers.

We had the most wonderful relationship with the press in the early days although, interestingly, one of the first mentions by a national newspaper columnist was double-edged. Veronica Papworth commented in the *Sunday Express*: 'Thank God Weight Watchers has come to England. Now fat people can bore each other, instead of boring the rest of us by talking about their diets at dinner parties.'

If using the media to spread the word was important, then so too was enlisting the support of the medical profession. During the late sixties obesity was considered to be a joke in England. Very few in the medical profession stood up to declare that obesity was a serious danger to health. Doctors in America were already warning the public about the risks of cholesterol, about hardening of the arteries, about heart disease — and their association with diet. Yet in Britain, doctors had not yet spelled out the many ways in which obesity could kill. No one explained that being fat increased the risks of surgery. No one had actually admitted that more people were dying from obesity than any other disease. The study of nutrition was not included in the average doctor's training. Children were taught nothing at school about healthy eating; they learned by copying what they saw at home, and frequently from the questionable meals served at school. The irony was that the generation which had been forced to eat properly, having lived through the war, was so resentful and weary of rationing that they wanted their children to have all the things they had been forced to do without. As a result they created the fattest, if not the most unhealthy, generation England had ever known. Later I was shocked to learn that the English consumed more chocolate per capita than any other country in the world.

Even when fat people went to their doctor for help to lose weight they were unlikely to come out of the consulting rooms or the surgery with anything really constructive. On the one hand there were the diet doctors who had rooms in Harley Street and offered expensive course of injections which were supposed to disperse fat, or who prescribed pills which hyped you up or suppressed your appetite. On the other, there were local GPs who simply handed out yet another diet sheet and a few words of warning or encouragement.

When Weight Watchers began people told us that — as lay people — we would run into stiff opposition from the medical profession. They also said that the profession in Britain was full of fuddy-duddies who were bound to resist anything new, particularly if it had come originally from America. But they were wrong, very wrong. We insisted that anyone with a medical problem of any kind had to obtain their doctor's consent before joining Weight Watchers. This way GPs soon became aware of who we were and what we were doing.

From the very beginning I sent copies of the Weight Watchers programme of eating to doctors throughout the country, as well as to experts in metabolism and nutrition. The replies we received applauded our work and approved the diet as a sensible one they could recommend. When other Weight Watchers heard the stories of the achievements of fellow members with severe medical conditions, they were further inspired to tackle their own, often less serious problems.

An Ealing member had joined Weight Watchers on the advice of her doctor. Unhappiness and worry about her weight had led to dangerously increased blood pressure and such a loss of self-confidence that she was considering giving up her job — her last link with the 'normal' world. As a personal assistant to a high-ranking civil servant, an important aspect of her work involved receiving visitors. As she became heavier, this became positive torture — she felt like 'a bus on legs'. She was no longer able to dress with any style, only too conscious that she no longer looked good in anything she wore. As a result she began making excuses to avoid visiting friends or inviting them to her own home. She became resigned to what then seemed inevitable: to adding an inch to her girth every year and eventually to being a little fat old woman — an appalling prospect.

A few days after passing her goal by 2 pounds, she wrote to tell me: 'Once again I can buy attractive clothes — I am confident, very active and unbelievably happy about it all. Your friendly understanding and comprehension of the difficulties that face us all gave me the courage to continue with the lectures and the Programme. I owe a lot of my present happiness to you.'

When Sandra Briggs, a handicapped member of the Streatham class, first joined Weight Watchers, she was unable to stand on the weighing machine, even with crutches, and had to be weighed on a chair placed across two machines and an allowance then made for the weight of the chairs and her leg irons.

Sandra was born with spina bifida. She was also a rather overweight baby, but as her life at that time consisted of hospital visits, either waiting to have an operation or recovering from one, for a long time the problem of her increasing weight was not tackled. As a teenager, a doctor put her on a diet which led to a weight loss of only 7 pounds in three months. Sandra came to the conclusion that to achieve the weight loss she really wanted, it might take three years and so her diet fell by the wayside.

Yet, nine months after a concerned neighbour had persuaded her to join a local Weight Watchers class, Sandra had shed an astonishing 5 stone (32 kilos) and could climb on to the scales unaided. From being the member who had to be aided and assisted by everyone, she became a class clerk and an inspiration to others.

For Sandra, as with so many of our disabled members or those with severe health problems, the most thrilling aspect of her weight loss was not the improvement in her medical condition but the fact that she could now wear hot pants! Time and again we saw people who were able significantly to increase their mobility because of weight loss — one man was even able to abandon his wheelchair — and yet when we asked them what was the most satisfying part of losing weight, we would be told it was the fact that for the first time they could buy their clothes off the peg, wear bright colours, take up one seat on a bus instead of two. In short, they had always seen their weight and not their disability as their principal problem.

A member of our Slough class had had osteoarthritis for a number of years, aggravated according to her doctor by overweight. Drastic measures were called for. She was hospitalized for a spell of intensive physiotherapy and weight reduction, but the hospital decreed the only way weight loss could be achieved was to cut down her food intake radically. She went on a strict regime of alternate days, one when she could eat 500 calories and one of complete starvation! After a painful, boring and very long time in hospital — fourteen and a half weeks in all — the operation took place and was pronounced a success. She was allowed to go home with some mobility restored to her previously crippled knees.

Needless to say, however, sticking to such a punitive dietary regime when not under medical supervision soon proved to be impossible, and to her despair the pounds started to creep back on, undoing the good effects of her operation. Soon she needed a stick to walk more than 20 yards, and going up and down stairs was a misery. A friend suggested Weight Watchers, her GP felt it could do no harm, and although at 13 st 7 lb (87 kilos) she at first felt the 9 st 2 lb (59 kilos) target was ridiculous, she also felt this was her last chance to avoid a miserable, crippled existence.

As her weight dropped to less than it had been in her teens, she began to feel 'wonderfully well — better than I have for about 10 years'. Losing weight didn't cure her arthritis but 'I can now walk quite a distance without my stick, get up and downstairs without it, and with it I can walk *and enjoy* a 2–3 mile hike — and unless you've been unable to do this, you've no idea what a joy it is.'

I began visiting local medical groups and was frequently asked to speak. Instead of finding the doctors disinterested and indifferent, I discovered they were welcoming and supportive. They all agreed that the failure rate for treating obesity within their practices was very high indeed and they were only too pleased to be able to unload the problem on to us. We sent all our successful members back to visit their GPs to show off. The doctors were impressed and soon they were sending us other patients.

As a result of this exercise, and because of our Bentall's fashion show, Weight Watchers was featured in an item on the BBC six o'clock television news. We were then inundated with more than 2,000 letters from people wanting to know where they could find a class near their home.

CHAPTER FOUR

Weight Watchers may have started off slowly but as we got rolling we were like a snowball, getting bigger and bigger all the time. In 1969 — two years after we began — Weight Watchers was registered as a limited company with a turnover of £29,000. The following year Weight Watchers lost over a million pounds — or at least our members did, in fat.

In February 1970 we opened our first class in Scotland; in April we opened in South Wales. The first class in Manchester had opened the previous year, but by November 1970 demand was so great in the North of England that we decided to open a regional office in Deansgate, Manchester, under the management of Pam Owen-Thomas. Pam, a trained barrister, had joined my original Datchet class in July 1967, and had gone on to become a lecturer and trainer. Now she was given the task of developing the northern area and by January 1971 there were more than 52 weekly classes in the northern counties alone.

People in the North seemed to have more serious weight problems. They waited so long for Weight Watchers to open in Manchester that when we did, 2,000 people showed up; we were forced to vacate the 'Lesser Hall', having been declared a fire hazard. I ended up lecturing in the street, begging people to come back the following week to register. Instead they waved their money in the air and insisted on joining there and then.

Doreen Rigby, then living in Windsor, had to be persuaded to make a weekly trip back to her childhood home in Manchester and teach classes there. She had enough new members to fill five classes immediately.

Another Weight Watcher who had to be persuaded to spread our gospel was May Angus. After thirty years as a widow she left Scotland to make a new life in England. I met her just after she had lost weight and qualified as a lecturer. I was desperate for someone to run our Scottish operation and finally convinced her.

In her sixties, she travelled hundreds of miles per month visiting and mothering all our lecturers and members. When I asked her to 'weigh in' people instead of animals at the Royal Highland Show, she, being a frugal Scot, rented a caravan (without a loo) for her Weight Watchers helpers. A retired antique dealer, Archie, was smitten by her and to show his devotion made her a gift of several antique 'potties' for the girls to use. Later he proposed that she retire with him and live in Wales.

The other supervisors and I gave her a farewell party in my home. She told us that there were three wishes she wanted more than anything — a haircut from one of Vidal Sassoon's salons, make-up lessons from Joan Price, Beauty Editor of *Harpers* magazine, and a chat with Fiona Richmond, who gave sex advice on late-night radio. I arranged to get them all there, particularly Fiona who came with Paul Raymond of the famous Raymond Revue Bar after her nightly show at midnight. How we all profited from her guidance!

Month by month Weight Watchers grew. In December 1970 there were 370 classes and a membership of just over 250,000. By the following June we had more than 450 classes and a membership which was fast approaching half a million. By the mid-seventies we had comfortably passed the million mark.

Mary Southall, our Welsh supervisor, was particularly innovative and daring. When the miners' strike broke out in 1974, toppling Edward Heath's government and almost paralysing the nation, I was determined not to close a single one of our 600 weekly classes. Without heat and light this was difficult, but not for Mary Southall. She organized a 'whip-round' and came up with enough miners' lamps to service all our classes. Within one weekend we had distributed supplies to our lecturers who ran romantic, lamplight meetings. Prince Philip was quoted as saying at that time, 'We are not afraid of Wedgwood Benn, but if these Weight Watcher ladies ever took it into their heads to take over the country — we'd be worried.'

Yet there were still millions more fat people in Britain for us to convert. Weight Watchers had certainly started something, but the eating habits of an entire nation were not going to change overnight.

Despite the terrible way most Americans ate, I was appalled when I really got to know the eating habits on this side of the Atlantic. I couldn't believe it when I saw people pouring double cream over cakes with whipped cream fillings — cream on cream. Britain is one of the few places in the world where this is still done.

Food was overcooked so that vegetables lost much of their nutritional value — the vitamins were thrown away with the water. Gravies and ketchups were used to disguise, rather than flavour, a meal. Meat always came with its own layer of fat (I used to get into trouble because I would ask for the fat to be cut off *before* the butcher weighed the meat). I had never seen silver and gold topped milk before. In America, all milk was homogenized. I even knew people, my husband included, who would drink only the top of the milk and pour the rest of the bottle away. The English were the only people who had spaghetti and chips — Italians never did.

Health was not a subject much discussed. Perhaps the greatest accomplishment of Weight Watchers was that it taught people the true dangers of obesity. It made them more aware of the importance of learning new eating habits and cooking skills. The preparation of meals could become more pleasurable if the process was made more creative and imaginative.

When I came to England in 1963 women shopped a day at a time. Few homes had refrigerators, so there was a storage problem. Frying was a common way of preparing foods, rather than grilling or poaching. I was amazed when I looked into other shopping baskets to see huge amounts of lard. Women made food go further by coating fish in a thick batter. People used to believe that when the weather was cold you needed stodgy, warming food. In the North many confided in me their certainty that fat was a protection against tuberculosis — sharing the same belief as my mother and her friends back in Brooklyn.

Many people still came home for lunch and had their main meal of the day then. We found it difficult to convince them of the merits of switching to a regime which meant eating more in the evening than at midday.

We believed that this was important because for most people their longest period of inactivity followed the evening meal. That was when people relaxed with a book or watched television. Our argument was that the metabolic rate was changed according to what you ate and when you ate it. Most people who went on a diet cut right down on food or didn't eat at all during the day — they seemed to feel an instinctive need to punish themselves by starvation. This was not only unnecessarily severe but also served to sabotage their metabolism. We taught that the body was like a furnace: in order to burn off all the excess fat you had to start the fire in the morning with a proper breakfast, you had to keep it going during the day by eating regularly, and stoke it up at night (when you were naturally less active) with a good meal. The choice, variety and volume of food had to be balanced nutritionally.

We also found it hard work to persuade men in particular to accept our total ban on alcohol. In a country where going to the pub for a few beers was part of the culture, keeping the no alcohol rule meant a great sacrifice. And as for chocolates — they were a part of life. No one seemed to go to the cinema or the theatre without their box of chocolates.

There was very little knowledge of or concern about nutrition. When I went to school in America in the fifties, we were taught what constituted a nourishing meal. Yet in England in the sixties there was little information available except that which was issued to young wives and mothers in pamphlets produced mainly by food manufacturers or other special interest groups. Baby-food manufacturers encouraged mothers to get their babies on to full-cream milk and fattening solids as soon as possible.

Even the technology was lacking. When I used the term a 'Teflon pan', people thought I was mad. Now non-stick pans are found in homes as a matter of course. In fact, what has happened in Britain's food habits has been truly revolutionary.

In the sixties people tended to see obesity as a condition to be treated lightly. Doctors advised individual patients that they needed to lose weight for the sake of their health or because surgery might be required and the fatter they were, the greater the risk of complications. Yet there were no government-funded health campaigns warning people of the dangers of being fat and, as a result, public awareness of the implications of obesity was almost non-existent. What Weight Watchers did was to re-educate people, and the effects were far-reaching.

One of our most important projects involved childhood and teenage obesity. We knew that eating patterns were usually established in childhood and carried on into adulthood; the fat child became a fat adult and was likely to have fat children — and so the cycle continued.

Since people of all ages joined Weight Watchers we had some young children in our classes and we knew how miserable they felt to be fat. Our youngest member was 6-year-old Robin Finesilver, who was 6st 5lb (41 kilos) when he joined our Hackney branch. That was pretty hefty for a boy of his age. The other children at Robin's school used to make fun of him and he hated sports and games because it meant undressing in the changing room in front of them. He would do anything to avoid gym, including pretending to be ill. Once he wrote a note to his teacher: 'Please excuse Robin from games today. He has a head-ache.' He signed it: 'Mummy'.

Robin did very well on our programme and lost a stone and a half in 16 weeks. But one of the main problems was caused by the school's attitude. Robin's mother wanted to send him to school with packed lunches to make it easier for him to stick to the programme, but the headmaster insisted that he eat school meals with the other children.

The school food was stodgy and fattening and it made things very difficult for Robin, who was doing his best. Even though Robin's mother implored the headmaster, he refused to accept that obesity was a problem in his school or to accommodate her son's needs.

I was furious when I heard about this because I knew that childhood obesity was a serious problem, not just in this school but in many others. I had been fat from the age of eleven, and well knew how overweight children could be humiliated. Therefore we encouraged Weight Watchers who had school-age children to approach head teachers to offer our services in measuring and weighing children in their schools. A number of heads agreed and we were able to prove that childhood obesity was, indeed, widespread and needed to be combatted.

It was at this point that I met Professor Arnold Bender who later became our nutritional adviser; he weighed into the debate with a statement on behalf of the Inner London Educational Authority saying there was no problem with that authority's school meals because they were carefully calculated to give each pupil the right calorie intake. His example was that if you had 150 children in a school, and each of them needed 'X' calories per meal, then the total amount of calories provided at the school dinner would be 'X' multiplied by 150.

This was fine in theory, but I knew things were different in practice and wanted to show the professor.

Together we visited a number of schools at dinner time, and in most cases everything went exactly as I predicted. Instead of dividing the food equally between the children, the dinner ladies dished out only about one-third during the first serving. This meant each child got less than his or her nutritional requirements. Next the ladies served up what remained to those children who came back for second helpings; these tended to be the fat children who came back for seconds, and for third and fourth helpings. Ruefully Professor Bender had to admit that there was a big gap between scientific theories and reality. He vowed to help us and proved to be a great asset and a valuable spokesman.

I was anxious to establish, as well, that school meals themselves bore no relation to anything resembling a balanced diet. There was far too much stodge and not enough fruit and vegetables to provide the vitamins, nutrients and minerals growing children needed. Puddings were always served with no choice of fruit as a substitute, and giving sweets as a reward was common practice at prize-giving ceremonies. On October 15th 1970 we held a press conference which discussed the problem of childhood obesity, and we launched our first class just for teenagers.

We found that a frightening number of children in Britain didn't have a proper breakfast — it simply wasn't an established family pattern. This surprised me because I had always thought the British were much better than the Americans about eating generally — not eating on the run, and having proper family meals. But this wasn't generally the case.

Our original idea had been to expand the number of classes for teenagers and younger children, holding them in schools wherever possible. Soon, however, we found that children didn't really want these classes in schools; they preferred a more friendly relaxed atmosphere. We also found that when children came to our ordinary Weight

Watchers classes they related very well to the older members, who were like grandparents to them. Often they would ring them during the week to talk — just as if they were truly related.

Within the family, too, it was often the grandparents who turned out to be better at teaching good eating habits to children than their parents were.

When a grandmother or a grandfather lost weight they usually became more active then they had been before, and therefore more involved with their grandchildren. They had the time and more patience and so they were a positive influence.

Of course, attitudes towards childhood obesity are different today. Health visitors are concerned when babies put on too much weight, rather than complimenting mothers on having such bonny, bouncing children, as in former days. School meals, however, still leave a great deal to be desired.

The medical profession's attitudes toward obesity have changed too, but hospital food is still dreadful. Often there remains that huge gap between theory and reality. We may have come a long way but there is still farther to go.

We passed perhaps the most important milestones for Weight Watchers during our first five years. Between 1967 and 72 there were other personal milestones — notably the birth to Richard and me of our third child, a daughter, Alesia, and almost simultaneously the publication of my first book, *The British Weight Watchers Cookery Book.*

Alesia was not the first Weight Watchers baby by any means. Her arrival on December 15th 1970 was announced in the national press under the headline: 'Bernice Weston loses a stone in one day — and they called her Alesia Hilarie Martine Weston'.

It was nice to think that whatever happened in Weight Watchers was newsworthy, but what pleased me most was that pregnant women and their doctors were beginning to take a different attitude towards childbearing. The old wives' tale about having to eat for two while pregnant was now becoming outdated. Weight Watchers taught that expecting a baby was, in itself, no reason to come off the Programme. We insisted that pregnant women consult with their doctors and follow any specific dietary advice they were given, but in most instances the medical advisers heartily recommended that overweight women continue to lose weight as long as they ate sensibly and wisely.

Many of our members continued to lose weight during their pregnancy and still produced 'bonny' babies. Jean Edwards, a member of the Morden class, weighed almost 14 st 5 lb (92 kilos) when she joined Weight Watchers. She became pregnant with twins. Even so, Jean weighed in at 11 st 4 lb after the birth of twins weighing 5 lb 2 oz and 5 lb 8 oz. She said she had never had such an uneventful pregnancy and such an easy delivery and that she felt healthier because she was on the Programme.

Alesia was born weighing a mere 6 lb 6 oz. My first child, Douglas, weighed 9 lb 13 oz (his size created complications for him and for me) and Graeme weighed 8 lb 8 oz. My own weight after Alesia's birth registered only 4 pounds above my goal weight of 8 st 8 lb (56 kilos)and only 8 pounds above my ideal weight of 8 st 4 lb (53 kilos).

Even so, I returned to class a few weeks after her birth, using my free lifetime membership. All during my pregnancy I had taken part in a control group of other pregnant Weight Watcher members. We monitored, as well as commiserating with, one another. My pregnancy had not been easy by any stretch of the imagination. Once again, I'd had thrombosis in my legs, and life was complicated by the fact that during the latter stages I was working flat out on an important new venture — my first cook book. In fact, if my smile appeared a little fixed in my photograph on the front cover of the book, it was because, heavily pregnant, I was propped up against the table, holding on to it, whilst the photographer took shot after shot.

There was great difficulty protecting the name of Weight

Watchers in the UK. Someone suggested we publish a book clearly connecting our approach and method with the name Weight Watchers. When Hamish Hamilton, the publishers, approached me to prepare a cook book for the United Kingdom, we agreed happily and proposed that we co-publish the book so that we could sell copies in our classes at a reduced price for our members. Because of the complications with my pregnancy, Richard wanted to defer this project until later, but I felt too committed to it to stop now. Richard organized a board meeting at which he and Leslie voted me down. Although I had the controlling shareholding I refused to use it as a veto. Instead, being headstrong and determined, I decided to publish the book myself.

I took my building society bank book to the office of Hamish Hamilton and asked him if he would accept my £10,000 savings (my only assets other than my interest in Weight Watchers) as surety for my commitment to purchase 50,000 copies for our classes. Hamish Hamilton was highly amused. Having published the works of some of England's most famous writers and personalities (he was then publishing the memoirs of Prince Philip), he admitted that this was a most unusual enterprise.

He pulled out all the stops to help me. Everyone seemed involved personally, even the manager of the printing firm, Sir Thomas Causton & Sons of Southampton. As soon as the first copy came off the presses he raced up to Windsor with his wife to present it as a newborn gift for Alesia. She was born two days later.

The British Weight Watchers Cookery Book sold — well, like hot cakes. It was reprinted just a month after publication. A year later it still topped the bestsellers list. Its success was due in part to the lavish colour illustrations which proved beyond doubt that menus which helped people lose weight and stay slim did not have to be boring or unappetizing. The very first photograph showed a pan of baked apples simply oozing raspberries; the soups looked warming; the salads exciting. The main courses were mouthwatering, and the puddings, which included soufflés and meringues, sumptuous. The illustrations were a visual banquet and proved beyond doubt that it was not necessary to feel deprived if you 'slimmed' by eating the Weight Watchers way.

I think Barbara Hardwick, Beryl Townsend, Gillian Rimmer and Louisa Pipe, like me, slept nary a night while this project was in progress. Our only immediate reward was to be able to taste the foods which we prepared for the photo sessions. If any of us was above goal weight we could only taste, not swallow. Carol McCartney, the Director of the Good Housekeeping Institute, saw that each recipe was tested until it was foolproof.

The book showed people how easy it was to serve 'legal' family meals or to give dinner parties that looked so lavish, no one would guess that the host or hostess was trying to lose weight.

We were also concerned to make it possible for our members to follow the Programme no matter where they ate or where they travelled. By this time forty restaurants throughout the country were serving Weight Watcher meals under licence from us, and in January 1971 British European Airways (BEA) began serving Weight Watcher meals on all their mainline flights.

I learned from many Weight Watchers, as I travelled through the country, that when they went abroad, holidays and business trips were threatening to their diet. As soon as they were offered their in-flight meal, which was tempting but fattening, they succumbed, lost their resolve and consequently fell from grace. Holidays thus became an invitation to disaster. I therefore approached BEA, who carried out extensive research and were surprised to learn how great was the demand among their customers for Weight Watchers meals. It took an entire year to organize everything but eventually the big day arrived and I was invited to inaugurate the project with a promotional flight to

Majorca. It was the first time anywhere in the world that an airline was to serve a Weight Watchers or slimming meal of any kind, and reporters and photographers eagerly surrounded me to publicize the story. You can imagine my excitement as I waited for the steward to bring me my tray — and my horror when I saw what was on it. After a year spent ironing out every last problem so that there would be no error, my beautifully arranged and perfectly 'legal' lunch arrived. It included, however, a tomato, which Weight Watchers at that time specifically excluded from lunchtime meals.

'Are you sure this is exactly the way this meal came on board?' I asked the steward. 'Oh, no,' he replied sweetly. 'I thought the tray needed some colour so I added something.'

Because of the success of these airline meals, Richard and I agreed that the time was now ripe to promote a variety of foods under the Weight Watchers label. Richard initiated discussions with a number of food manufacturers as well as with the forward-looking supermarket chain Tesco.

No matter how diversified Weight Watchers became, the structure of the individual classes remained the same. There were a number of rules about the way classes were run. For instance, we never disclosed how much a person weighed. That was a secret between the lecturer (or the weigher) and the member. All we ever discussed was how much each member lost, and we applauded even half-pound losses.

It became clear that there were interesting differences between American and English women. Americans think they are honest, frank and outspoken but appearances can be deceptive. For instance, American women tend to slice a few years off their age. English women, by contrast, don't seem to mind telling their true age, whatever it may be. When it comes to weight, Americans follow a similar pattern. One American Weight Watcher told me that when a state trooper stopped her for a traffic offence and asked to see her driving licence, he looked at her height and weight entries and asked her if she had been ill (she had falsified her licence by knocking off 70 pounds from her weight).

Our English Weight Watchers showed no shyness or sensitivity about being weighed in public. One woman, a headmistress of a famous girls' school, when weighing in for her Weight Watchers badge, a pin with diamante chips for each 10 pounds lost, told me she had 'braved all the elements'. What she meant was that in mid-winter she had arrived without any underclothes or hosiery just to earn another 'chip'.

The American woman is casual, almost careless in her dress. Our English Weight Watchers came groomed and . dressed up as if each meeting was a very important social occasion.

Unlike their American counterparts, British women had very few opportunities to share intimate feelings and personal thoughts with others. Weight Watchers provided just such a forum. Once someone had shared a personal revelation, the lecturer would use this to elicit responses from other members, linking their problems to this situation. At the meetings we would discuss why we ate, and frequently we found that we were unhappy at home, felt inadequate about work, had a mother-in-law who made our lives a misery, were worried about our children or felt sexually unattractive. All kinds of problems were revealed when a member confessed to cheating: perhaps a woman would admit she was facing a divorce or that a parent was dying, and as usual food became her only solace. The other group members would band around her and offer her true comfort and understanding. I was fond of telling journalists, psychiatrists and therapists that Weight Watchers was not merely a weight-loss organization in the United Kingdom. Frequently the sharing that took place in class brought about new friendships and practical solutions to other problems of living.

For instance, in the Datchet class one week, I asked one woman why she had succumbed and gained weight after such a brilliant start. She explained that she was the mother of a child with Down's syndrome; whenever she or her husband became ill she began to worry what would happen to their child after their death, since they had no immediate family. At the end of the meeting I watched another member put her arm around her and the two women left together. The next week my errant member explained that the other member also had a Down's syndrome child; she explained how she and her husband attended a special holiday home in which handicapped children were made to feel welcome. She explained further that through an insurance policy the child would be able to live at this home permanently if the parents died.

'That way,' she explained, 'we know that if anything happens to us, our child will have a place in a home with people she already knows, with all the financial arrangements covered.'

What was amazing to me was that in this small village two mothers were facing the same kind of problem and yet they had never communicated before. For me, bringing these two together was one of the most valuable achievements of Weight Watchers in Britain.

British women, given a novel opportunity to share, frequently unburdened themselves of their fear of disease — especially cancer. Because of this fear many of our members were afraid to go for cervical smear tests. I was amazed to hear people tell me that in all cases that they knew of cancer victims, the patient died. I discovered that the women who had cancer and recovered never spoke of it, as if it were a stigma. And so the myth persisted that cancer was fatal. Our lecturers agreed to tackle this problem by using their own life experiences with this disease and to encourage others to speak openly.

If we helped to alter attitudes to cancer and other physical diseases we also altered people's attitudes to depression, stress, anxiety and mental breakdowns — we lessened the stigma of mental illness by the sharing of personal stories.

It is perhaps not stretching the analogy too far to say that in the early days of Weight Watchers we were confronting many of the same issues and using many of the same techniques as the emergent feminist movement with their 'consciousness raising'. No doubt diehard feminists will throw up their hands in horror at this — after all, in the words of Susie Orbach's book on the subject, to them *Fat Is A Feminist Issue* — but if ever anyone tried to tell me that in losing weight my members were mindlessly conforming to male-imposed stereotypes of female desirability, I had only to refer them to the often amazingly moving and poignant testimony of our members on what their weight loss had meant to them.

Certainly in some cases it was something as 'trivial' as being able to buy a dress or a trouser suit stock size instead of hiding away beneath custom made tents — though try telling an ex-26-stone (165 kilo) fatty that her achievement in slimming to a size 14 dress size is mindless conformism and you'll get a pretty dusty answer! In terms of her own increased self-confidence and sense of self-worth, that woman's achievement is no less negligible than that of her fellow dieter whose weight loss is the trigger to sort out an unsatisfactory home situation or apply for a new job.

In so many cases weight loss was merely the first step in a series of life-enhancing changes for successful Weight Watchers 'graduates'. Women went on quite literally to change their personality, outlook, expectations, family dynamics, employment prospects, in short their *lives*, because they had made that vital first step of taking control of their own body's craving for the solace and escape that food offered them. And it wasn't just their own attitudes they changed. When we first started, for instance, several of my lecturers had difficulty in opening a special account in which to bank their Weight Watchers takings. As married women, they were told by their bank managers that they would need their husband's permission to do this. I went in to bat on their behalf and in every case this absurd stipulation, left over from the previous century, was waived.

I was and am overwhelmingly proud of the achievements of the women (and men) we worked with in Weight Watchers. Yes, the feminist movement did lead to significant steps forward in a woman's right to control her own destiny — but I believe that the work of Weight Watchers and the achievements of its members, starting as early as 1967, helped to start the ball rolling.

It became terribly important to be honest at meetings, not only about your weight but about everything. We all confessed at these meetings about our attitudes towards fat, our deceitfulness about bingeing and cheating on diets.

Members supported each other through all kinds of crises with the lecturer frequently in the lead, acting as a catalyst, and helped to raise money for local charities through sponsored slims, fashion shows and other events. The Weight Watcher class became an important part of the fabric of the local community.

I suppose that the reason our groups worked so well was because we shared one important common denominator: 'fat'. Because of our rule that only people with at least 10 pounds to lose were eligible for membership, no casual slimmers or little starlets who wanted to lose a pound or two were admitted, and hence our overweight members could let down their guard. The rule applied no matter who you were.

Once the actress Miriam Karlin wanted to join. She had come to us just after she had been to a health spa and having lost weight did not have the requisite 10 pounds to lose, so we turned her away. The lecturer asked me to ring her to explain and when I began talking she interrupted: 'That's all right, I've been back a week and I've already gained the weight now, so I am eligible to join.' And join she did, and became an inspiration — as amusing and

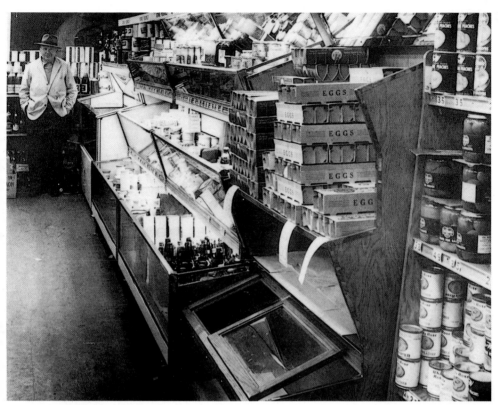

'If I had my life to live over, I'd live it over a grocery store.' Morris Turkewitz in his grocery store, Brooklyn.

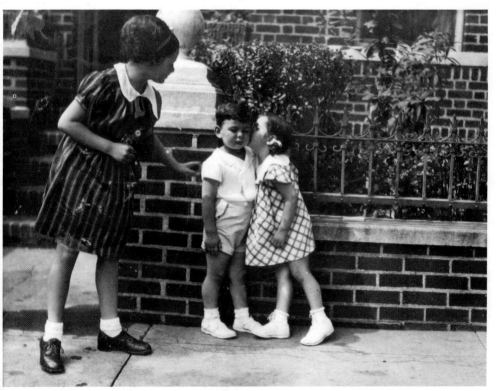

In Brooklyn all is love and kisses – Bernice with Solly Zaltman, while sister Diana looks on.

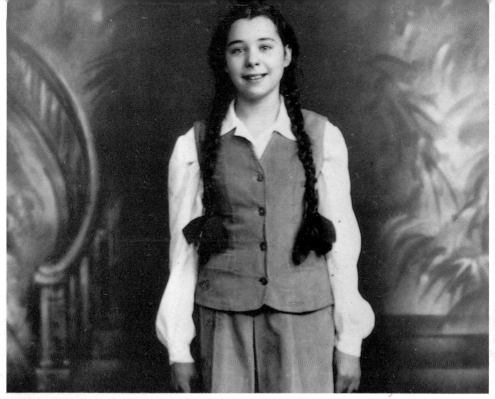

Bernice, aged 11, before a broken leg started her weight gain.

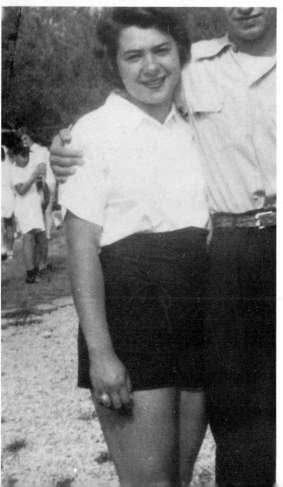

Bernice sighs about her thighs.

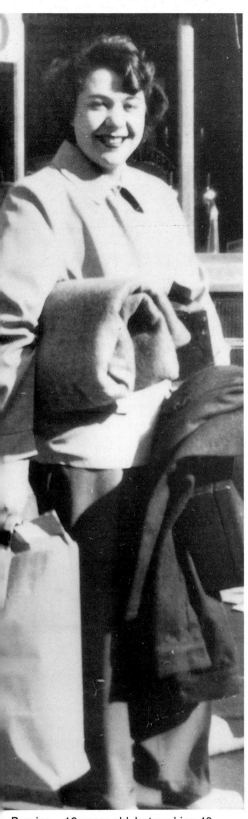

Bernice – 16 years old, but pushing 40.

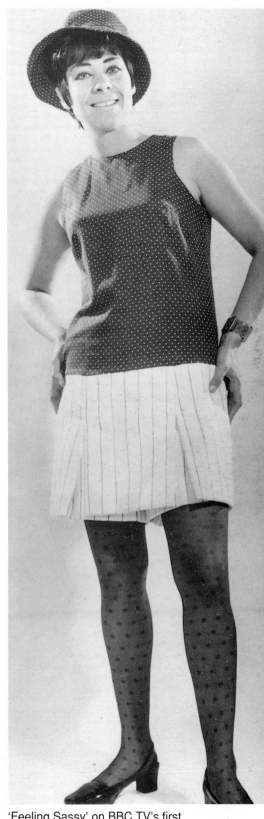

'Feeling Sassy' on BBC TV's first appearance.

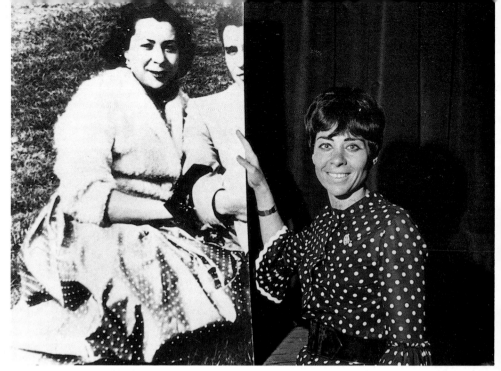

'See you lighter' – the fat girl in a size 10.

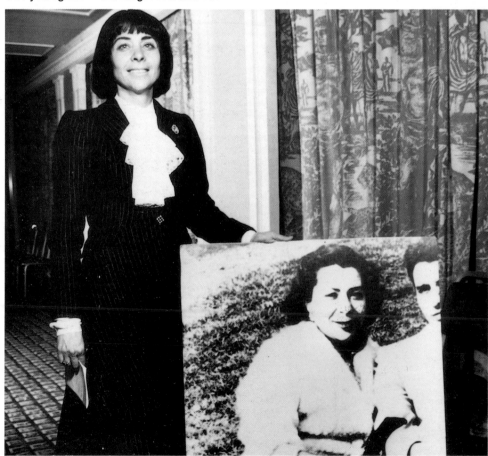

Through thick and thin – guess which one is pregnant?

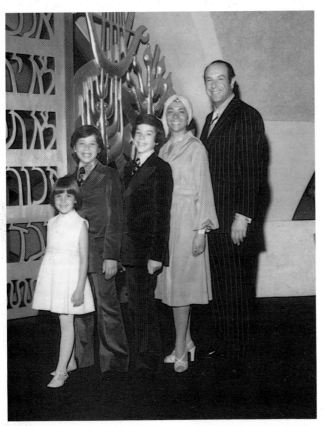

The Weston family celebrate (from right to left): Richard, Bernice, Douglas the Bar Mitzvah boy, Graeme and Alesia.

Matching sizes and styles with Katie Boyle.

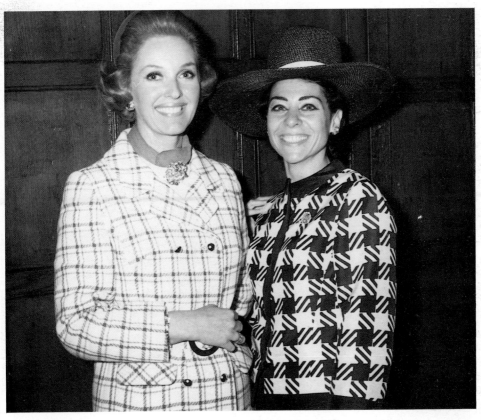

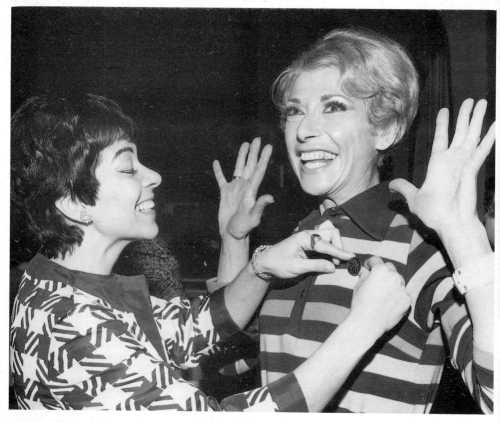

'My turn to laugh' – Miriam Karlin receiving her Weight Watchers pin.

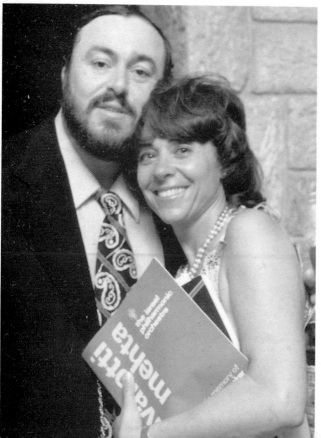

Singing for his supper – Pavarotti's slim–in with Bernice.

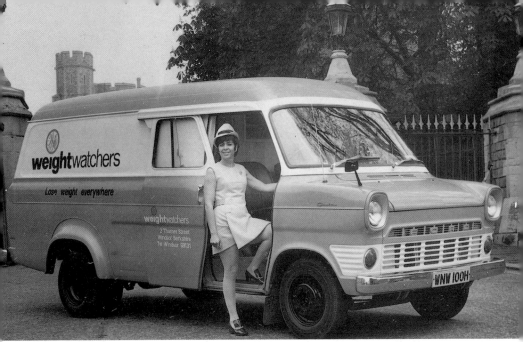

'Lose Weight Everywhere' – a royal occasion for Weight Watchers' first van.
Photo © Middlesex and Bucks Picture Service.

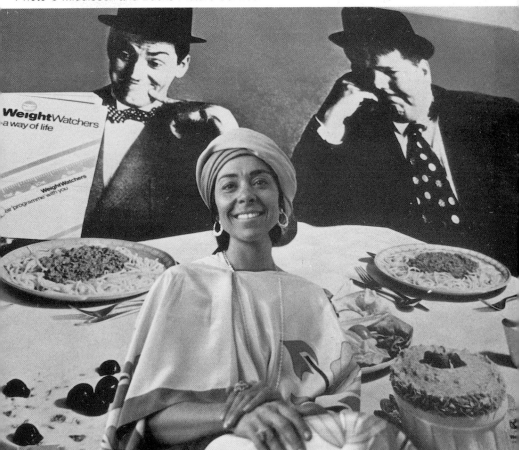

'I chose the souffle' – Bernice on the publication of her third cookbook.
Photo © Northcliffe Newspapers Group Ltd.

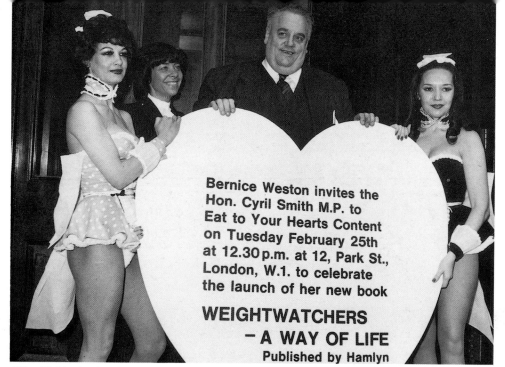

Bernice Weston invites the Hon. Cyril Smith M.P. to Eat to Your Hearts Content on Tuesday February 25th at 12.30 p.m. at 12, Park St., London, W.1. to celebrate the launch of her new book

WEIGHTWATCHERS – A WAY OF LIFE

Published by Hamlyn

'Slim Pickins' – the Right Honourable Cyril Smith receives a book invitation from Bernice on Valentine's Day. *Photo © HJH Design Services Ltd.*

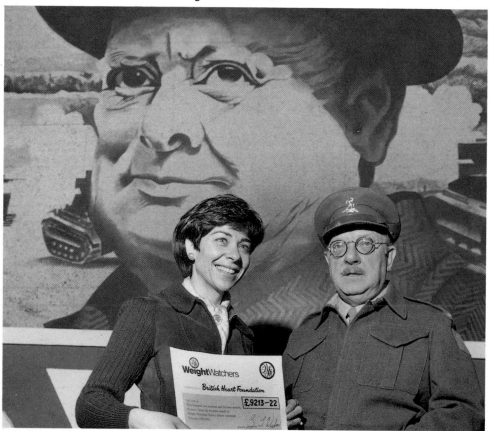

Churchill, 'Dad's Army' and Weight Watchers – three Great British institutions. *Photo © Raymond G.F. Nicholls.*

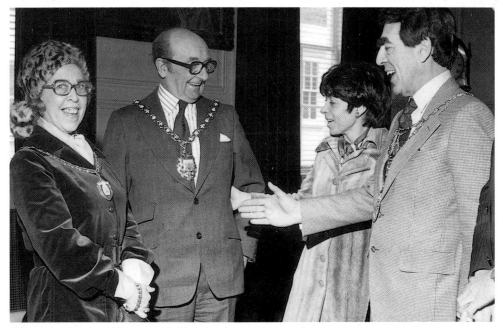

Kit Aston, Mayor of Windsor (right), after losing 3 stone for charity.
Photo © Raymond G. F. Nicholls.

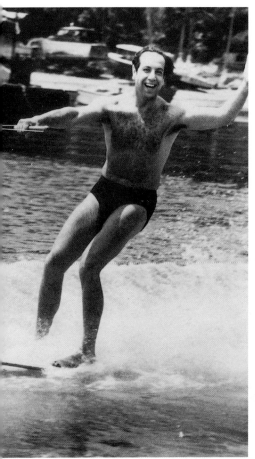

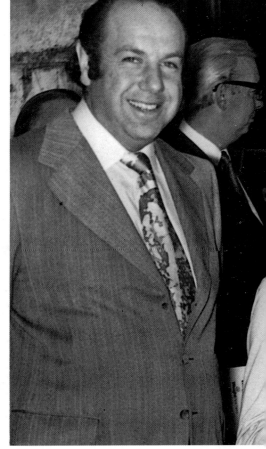

Richard Weston before and after – only in reverse.

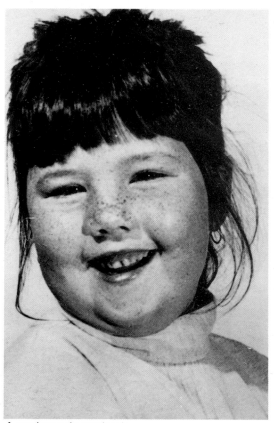
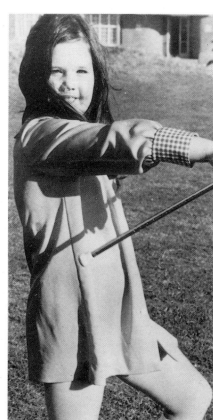

A modern minor miracle.

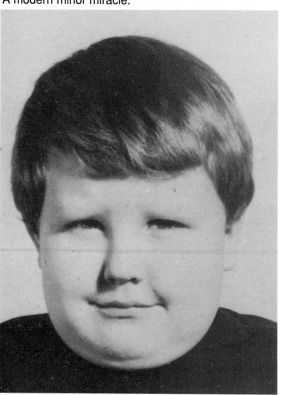
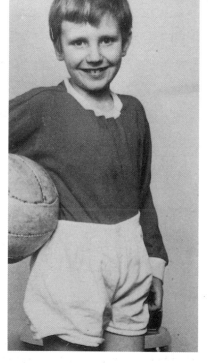

Modern miracle for a minor.

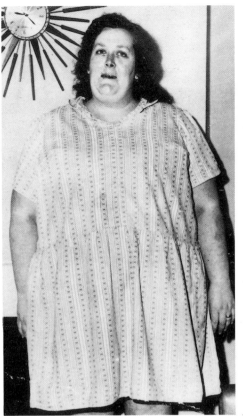
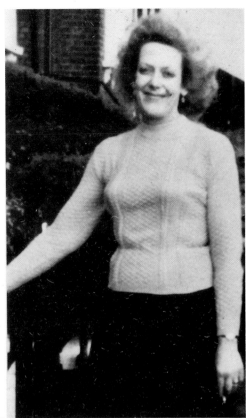

'No belly price' – Dolly Wager lost 20 stone in 20 months.

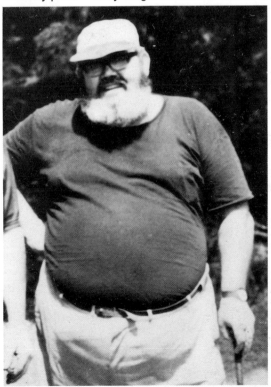
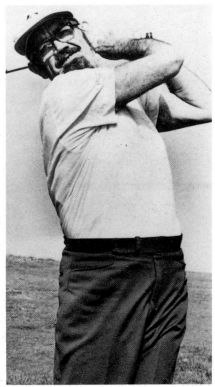

'How to improve your swing' – George Eaton loses 13 stone.

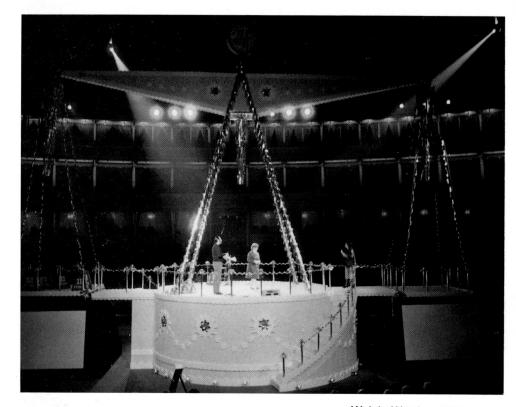

Evening Standard

45,880   London: Saturday January 8 1972   2   4p

Weight Watchers' fifth birthday party at the Albert Hall took London by storm.
Photo © Cryer & Marchant Ltd.

Weight Watchers jam London

A MASS rally of the U.K. members of an expanding international organisation was being held this evening in London's Royal Albert Hall. Those attending, all remarkably slim and healthy looking, had gathered to celebrate an unusual phenomenon.

They had all lost weight in varying amounts and had maintained their respective weight losses for periods of time ranging from five years in respect of earlier members and two to three months in respect of some more recent converts.

Few organisations can boast that their success is dependent on losses and even fewer on maintaining those losses year after year.

Six thousand members descended on the Albert Hall to hear their leaders talk of plans for the future. And they were joined by radio and television links — by thousands more who were unable to get to London.

Forward to Wembley in '73

GOOD EVENING Ladies and Gentlemen. When we said that in 1967 it w a s inappropriate because there were only three ladies and no gentlemen. Tonight there are 6000 of us gathered here at the Royal Albert Hall and our main regret is that we have had to refuse and turn away so many thousands of people—Weight Watchers and members of the public alike—who have asked for tickets.

Does this mean that we should book Wembley Stadium for 1973. Will the Cup Final have to be postponed?

Look out World, here we come. Basically that is what we said in 1967 and here we are. I think every one of us can take considerable pride in being here tonight because we are in the forefront of a major social battle and that needs no further explanation because we all know what I mean. But it is not inappropriate, but not entirely necessary, for me to congratulate and thank the lecturers, clerks, weighers, supervisors and Head Office Staff of the Weight Watchers organisation numbering several hundred who are with us tonight. They know from themselves and from you the value of their own achievement.

You, too, can be proud not only of your achievement for yourselves but of the example you have set to people yet to become members, some people who had it not been for you and your success perhaps would not have joined and would have gone on suffering.

Traffic built up steadily throughout London during the afternoon until by 5 o'clock the A.A. and R.A.C. joint spokesman announced from the Ministry of Transport, that the situation was no longer under control.

Jams stretched throughout East Anglia, Kent, Sussex, Buckinghamshire, Berkshire and Middlesex and most streets in the Home Counties had come to a standstill.

Jams were reported on all motorways and cross Channel ferry services were stopped to prevent a further influx of excited enthusiasts from the Continent.

BANNED

A BEA spokesman indicated that Heathrow was now controlled by the Royal Air Force and all incoming flights had been banned. Another airline said their services around the world would be disrupted as a direct result of being unable to get aeroplanes away from Heathrow, but they hope to be back to normal next week. Pan American and TWA announced that they would over-fly London during the occupation.

The Cabinet was in session from late last night and a communiqué from 10 Downing Street this morning said that rumours of a Coalition Government to cope with the crisis were totally unfounded.

The Leaders of the Opposition and Liberal Parties announced that they would in any event, stand by.

A Scotland Yard spokesman announced that no estimated 1,500,000 people had camped out in Hyde Park and Kensington Gardens during the night and the Red Cross had been flying in supplies by helicopter.

In Kensington Gardens was to be turned into a helicopter evacuation base.

In Windsor, Berkshire, home town of the headquarters of the Weight Watchers organisation, the story was different. All seemed calm and the people

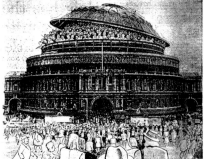

Jams spread to Lancashire. The scene on the M4 at noon today

went about their daily business as usual.

A spokesman for the Weight Watchers organisation said that as far as they were concerned, the situation was no different than any other day and a team of supervisors and lecturers were dealing with the situation and deal with any emergencies as they arise. Director Mr. Leventon had gone home early to change in readiness for the evening festivities and was unable to comment.

As our supplies were flown into the London area by lorries the word went out from the Weight Watchers London Control Centre: Civilians and children first !

The Government Emergency Committee spokesman admitted that he expected things to be back to normal by Wednesday of next week and there was a suggestion of setting up a Committee to investigate any further plans by the Weight Watchers organisation for future plans of this nature.

It seems that this organisation holds a serious threat to peaceful over-indulgence. The war on obesity is taking hold.

Weight Watchers raise the roof at the Albert Hall

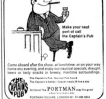

Make your next port of call the Captain's Pub

Come aboard after the show, at lunchtime, or on your way home any evening, and enjoy our nautical specials, draught beers or tasty snacks in breezy, maritime surroundings.

The Captain's Pub, Normal Pub hours
The Captain's Galley: Casual meals 24 hrs a day

Arrive at The **PORTMAN** way for good

PORTMAN SQUARE, LONDON W1. 01-486 5844

More pictures and news on Back Page

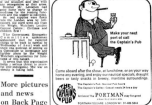

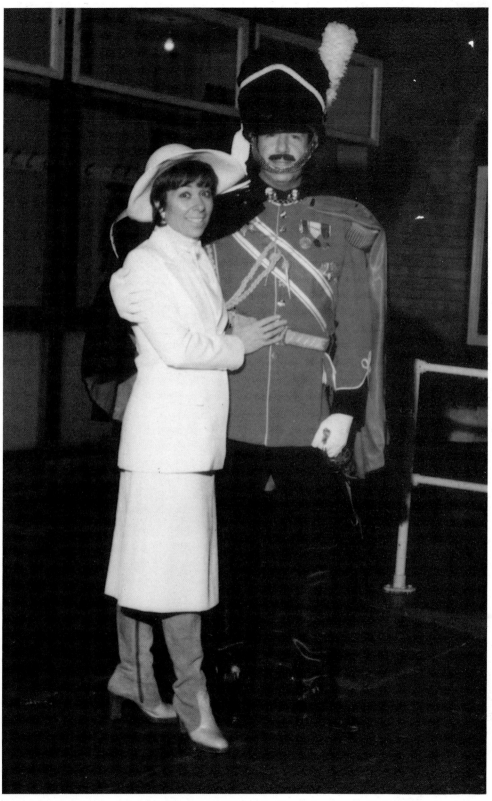

A royal messenger celebrating Weight Watchers' tenth anniversary – Richard Weston in disguise – it certainly fooled his wife!
Photo © Raymond G. F. Nicholls.

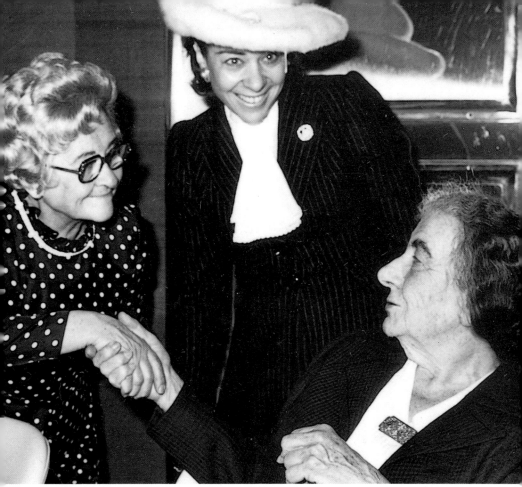

Mother Celia Turkewitz and Golda Meir – both originally from Pinsk – celebrating with Bernice in Israel.
Photo © Sidney Harris

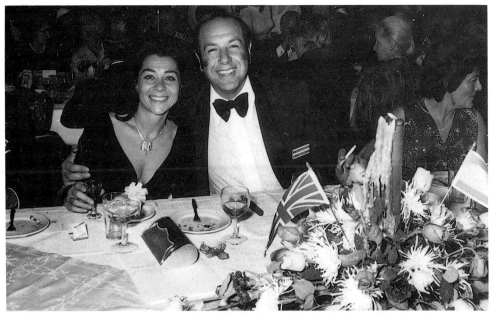

Before the fall – Bernice and Richard celebrate book, baby and birthday.

From: The Rt. Hon. Edward Heath, M.B.E., M.P.

HOUSE OF COMMONS

20th August, 1974.

Dear Mr Bilton,

Mr. Heath has asked me to thank
you for sending him the material and
excellent recipes which your Association
produces.

As you can imagine he has asked me
to say that his feelings were somewhat
mixed about doing so well in this
particular election!

Yours sincerely,

William Waldegrave
Private Office
Leader of the Opposition

N. B. Bilton, Esq.

The Right Honourable William Waldergrave, present Minister of Health but then assistant to Edward Heath, thanks Weight Watchers for the dubious honour bestowed on the Leader of the Opposition.

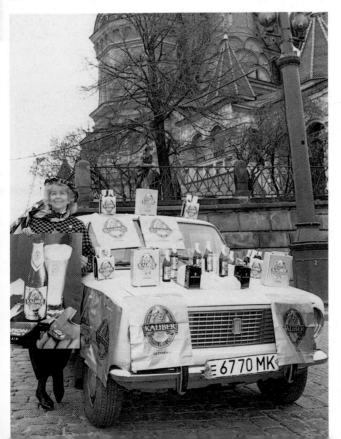

'Guinness Stout, Guinness Lean' – Bernice promoting low–calorie Kaliber with a display in Kremlin Square, Moscow.

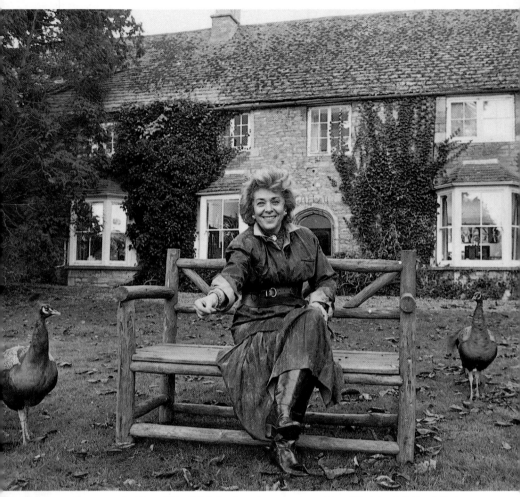

Bernice relaxes at Ashton, WiseWeighs headquarters – with a Weight Off Her Mind.
Photo © Northamptonshire Evening Telegraph.

delightful in the class as she was on the screen.

We never talked about how much weight a member had to lose. Instead we talked about learning how to eat properly. We used to tell people that if they wanted to join in order to be a size 12 for their daughter's wedding, they should think instead whether they wanted to be size 12 for their granddaughter's wedding. That was Weight Watchers' goal.

And we certainly didn't talk about calories (although the basic diet for women was approximately 1,200 calories a day) any more than we talked about fats or carbohydrates or protein. We talked about meals — breakfast, lunch and dinner, with in-between snacks — and food: bread, fish steaks and broccoli. Our view was that people don't eat calories or carbohydrates, they eat food at mealtimes. That was also why we talked about fat people, not obese people. Obesity was a medical term, fat was real.

One lesson I learned the hard way was that unless a fat person has made a real commitment to lose weight there is no point in lecturing or criticizing. The only time you can help is when they actually ask for help. If they don't then there is nothing you can do. In fact, anything you do try is more likely to have a negative result. When a fat person does want to lose weight, it is best pursued not by turning to the family, to a husband or wife, but to similarly afflicted people who can offer appropriate understanding and group support. Most of us learned that our husbands or wives, however sympathetic, were not qualified or attuned enough to be much help. In fact the very relationship is often counterproductive; it is like a husband teaching his wife to drive.

From my own experience I made the point that a wife should never try to be a lecturer to her husband. The relationship is too close and intense. That role needs to be played by a professional — and a Weight Watchers lecturer is a true 'professional'.

To ensure that my lecturers always performed as such, I made sure they were supplied with lecture themes and fresh material they could use to motivate their members. I went through newspaper cuttings, magazines, medical journals, and sought information and ideas from doctors, nutritionists, psychiatrists, psychologists and other health experts, which the lecturers could then share with their groups.

Although the classes dealt with serious problems, humour was a tool we used effectively. Obesity was referred to as 'food in mouth disease'. Weight Watchers was called the 'Court of Weights and Measures'. We enjoyed poking fun at the 'skinnies' — after all, we had suffered enough jokes about 'fatties'.

We all had a lot of fun. But the real satisfaction lay in knowing we were helping people, some of whom had begun to think of themselves as beyond help. Only once in Weight Watchers did we doubt our ability to rise to the occasion.

One day a lecturer received a call from a London doctor who asked if he could refer a patient who was suffering from severe heart trouble. His patient was advised that unless she lost weight she might only have six months to live. The woman, who weighed 50st 2lb (319 kilos) was in such a desperate state that she was driven from her Brixton flat to the class in an ambulance, bringing her own chair and carrying a supply of oxygen, in case of an emergency.

The lecturer was frightened and felt out of her depth. She called me for advice and I telephoned the doctor to explain, politely, that this was one situation which was too complicated for a lay group like Weight Watchers. 'That's all right,' said the doctor, 'but you must understand that you've just sentenced this woman to death.'

What could we do? And that was how Jean Renwick, who was recorded in the *Guinness Book of Records* as Britain's largest woman, joined Weight Watchers — and possibly saved her life.

CHAPTER FIVE

Jean turned out to be very personable and bright and the class adored her. At first she was motivated purely by the desire to stay alive, but as the pounds and then the stones began to drop off, and she no longer faced a life-or-death situation, we realized we would need to find other ways of encouraging her to carry on to her goal weight.

First we discovered that she wanted to learn to drive — so she needed to lose enough weight to get behind the wheel of a car. Then she wanted to be able to go to the hairdresser, so she had to lose more weight in order to be able to fit into the chair in the salon. Her next ambition was to learn to swim. Then it was to be able to wear clothes she didn't have to make for herself. Each time she reached one of her goals, we were able to find another to keep her motivated.

Jean was an extreme example, but in many ways she was also typical of our members. From her, we learned the importance of giving people new motives for continuing to lose weight. As their figures changed they became, quite literally, new people.

For me, one of the great advantages of Weight Watchers was that I was constantly on show. This motivated me to stay slim. I had to set an example to my lecturers, clerks, supervisors and members: I felt it would be letting them down if my weight went up again and that imposed a tremendous obligation on me.

Of course there were inevitably times when temptation in one form or another simply proved too much for people — but we used to warn our members that there was a good chance their sins would find them out. One of the incidents of cheating which became famous in Weight Watchers was both hilarious and moving. A Weight Watcher who had lost over 7 stone (45 kilos) went on holiday to Canada to visit her brother. She was admonished by her lecturer to join a Weight Watchers class there as quickly as possible, utilizing her free lifetime membership which was recognized all over the world by the Weight Watchers organization. Unfortunately she did not take advantage of this opportunity and, in fact, tempted by all the new foods in this 'foreign land', put back 3 of the 7 stone she had lost. She decided when she returned to her home that she would not rejoin Weight Watchers immediately but would find a job in another city, lose weight on her own, and then return with no one the wiser about her weight gain. She went for several interviews and was rejected at all of them. After her last job interview she felt tired and depressed and decided to cheer herself up with a cup of hot coffee.

At the self-service counter her eye ran over all the delights on display — sandwiches, cakes, and last of all her greatest weakness: doughnuts. She was tempted to cheat, as she explained when she told us the story, but the words of her fellow dieters and lecturer rang in her ears and she forced herself to walk past, determined not to weaken. At the end of the counter she ordered a cup of coffee and sat down at an empty table. A man asked if he could share her table and sat down with a tray which, to her horror, revealed a cup of coffee and a plate bearing two doughnuts.

Thinking bitter thoughts about Weight Watchers and the Programme, she looked the other way as he bit into the first bun. While she was still dwelling on her misery the man suddenly got up and left; she saw to her delight that he had left one doughnut behind on his plate. Surely God had taken pity on her and sent this as a message of solace and love. She was tempted, took the doughnut off the plate, and just as she was happily biting into it she looked up; to her horror the man reappeared at the opposite side of the table with a second cup of coffee! Unable to think sensibly about what to do she stood up, screamed, and ran from the restaurant. Later she called her lecturer and we all shared not only the humour of the situation but her ultimate success when she returned to goal. Weight Watchers all over the world have shared this story which moved us to laughter and to tears. We understood that the true moral was that our classes provided a real home to return to when in trouble; there was no scolding — only acceptance and loving understanding. The number of endorsements I received from grateful Weight Watchers graduates are a moving testimony to this.

One north London woman, for instance, wrote me a heartfelt letter of thanks after reaching her target weight of 10 stone. (64 kilos) 'At the rate I was going I fully accepted (and expected) that by the time I had been married 20 years, I would weigh 20 stone. I have recently celebrated my 20th anniversary weighing exactly half what I anticipated. My husband wants to say thank you for giving him his original wife back. Thank you again for everything you have helped me to do for myself. You have always been an inspiration to me. (I even have your likeness stuck to the lid of the cake tin!)'

One of the things I always insisted on right from the very start of Weight Watchers was that members who needed help in between classes should be able to ring their lecturer. It was far better to call for help than to cheat. Families often helped prevent cheating too. The teenage daughter of one member was so cross when she caught her mother guiltily about to bite into a biscuit one afternoon that she took the tin away, locked it in a wardrobe and refused to hand over the key.

Another woman used to find it hard not to cheat when she was invited out to coffee mornings. She told her husband that when people offered her cakes she didn't like to offend them by saying no.

His response was to tell her to eat all the cakes she

wanted — and he would make sure her tombstone was inscribed, 'She didn't like to offend.'

People joined Weight Watchers for many different reasons. New members were always asked what had brought them to the class. The answers were as varied as our members. Some mentioned their children, who became ashamed of having a fat mother or father as they grew up. Others said their children had asked them not to come to school speech day or sports day, because they didn't want to be seen with them.

One of the funny stories we used to tell was about a little girl who, when asked what she wanted to be when she was as big as her mother, replied in all seriousness, 'On a diet'. But all too often that kind of remark was wounding.

Men frequently said they had joined for medical reasons or because they were frightened when one of their friends keeled over and died from a heart attack. Women were more likely to say they hated the way they looked. One recalled the day she considered buying herself a pair of Capri pants — until her husband remarked that Capri was an island, not a continent.

The first man who joined us was one of our friends, Gordon Rose, who weighed in at almost 19 stone (121 kilos). Gordon was so fat you could hear him puffing and panting before you saw him. He had problems with his chest and problems with his feet, and because he was an engineer who had to carry out site inspections, his insurance company had loaded his premiums because they said he was so overweight he wasn't safe on a ladder.

Gordon, who performed the 'three-suit striptease' act at our Bentall's fashion show, gained in confidence as he lost weight and actually trained one of our lecturers.

Peter Eatwell, an architect, was another of our very early members. Peter was worried that at Weight Watchers he would find himself the only man in a room full of menopausal women, but I managed to reassure him enough for him to come to his first class. Giving up alcohol was one of his biggest challenges because he said that clients felt uncomfortable having a drink unless he kept them company. I told him that no one really cared what was in anyone's glass but their own, and there was no reason why he couldn't drink so long as it was tomato juice or soda water.

Peter lacked confidence until he lost 5 stone. Then he marched in and asked for a more senior position in his firm, something which he would never have dared to do before. He taught me something very important about the way fat people see themselves — even after they have lost weight. Some time after he had slimmed down he was sent a promotional leaflet by the outsize shop where he used to buy all his suits. He was furious that anyone should think he needed to shop there. But old habits died hard: on the very same day he had an appointment to see a doctor for an examination in connection with an insurance policy. The doctor told him he was in great shape, but during the examination Peter hesitated to walk between two chairs — demonstrating what an obstacle the outdated image of himself he carried in his head still was.

It is true that after people lose large amounts of weight they still carry around a mental image of themselves as very large. You have to change their view of themselves, and you have to change their family's view of them, too, so that they no longer continue to give them large helpings at every meal.

Oddly enough, losing weight can be very unnerving for someone who has been fat all their life. If you are a fat teenager you miss out on a whole area of development — the time when you experiment with your appearance and learn how to present yourself. If you are fat you go out of the way not to drawn attention to yourself: you wear dark colours, you avoid fabrics like wool, which clings. Going shopping for clothes is a nightmare — it's the time when you have to face up to the truth about how much weight you have put on; nothing fits and the sales girl is always overly sympathetic. And even when you have lost weight, you still tend to hang on to all your old ways. Shopping is always onerous — more like a punishment.

When I was a teenager my mother used to take my sister off late-night shopping and buy all my clothes for me. It was a family joke. They would come home, wake me up, try things on me and I never really knew what was going on, except that the next day there was a brand-new outfit for me to wear.

This made it easier for me later — even though I was slim — to let Richard shop for many of my clothes. He used to take some of my things to designers so that they knew what size I was and then have them make up outfits for me to wear.

Buying make-up was a mystery for many formerly fat people. When I was still fat I always bought Mary Quant make-up, not just because the counter was closest to Harrods Food Hall, but also because it was tucked away in a corner where no one could observe you if you wanted to try out a new lipstick or eyeshadow.

During our classes it emerged that many women felt exactly the same way. They never volunteered to have a free facial or make-up demonstration. They never ever wanted to be in the spotlight.

Because of this, many formerly fat people had little clothes sense or experience with make-up. Some women came to the class wearing the same old faithful dresses — while others went completely over the top in the other direction. I remember meeting one lecturer who was wearing a mini skirt so short I thought she would get arrested.

Soon it became clear that we needed to help people come to terms with their new selves, to lose the habits they had acquired when they were fat and to start acting and thinking like the thin people they now were. The very first fashion show at Bentall's had indicated how hard it was for people to change their old self-image — and how wonderful they could look once they knew how to make the best of themselves and had gained in self-confidence. Now the feedback from classes confirmed how crucial this step was.

It was for this reason that I decided to remake myself and

take along with me those of my lecturers who were also prepared to try. We called in Joan Price of the Face Place and she let us come to her studios and play like little children. We all shared a total dislike of the acid-tongued teenagers who stood behind the counters at Boots' make-up counters, being so competent and smart and making us feel so inadequate.

Weight Watchers encouraged couples to learn to do things they had never done before in their social life such as taking dancing lessons. Many couples did not dare go out dancing because they felt that a fat couple would look ridiculous. We also encouraged them to make things with their hands — to keep busy doing creative things rather than merely eating. Having an end product, which they could show off with pride, proved to be uplifting.

Many of the members were thrilled with the changes in themselves. Pat Brown — the woman who had to be weighed in on the luggage scales at Victoria Station — gave an interview to the *Daily Mail* after she had slimmed down from 27 to 13½ stone (172 kilos to 86 kilos). In the interview she said, 'Every day so many little things remind me how wonderful it is to be this new me. I can wear ordinary shoes now; before it had to be men's lace-ups. I can pick up things that I drop — before I had to wait for my husband or daughter to come home and do it. I've started wearing make-up — there never seemed any point before because no one looks at a face when there is a huge body to stare at.

'But it's the mental change that is really marvellous. It's the first time I've had a personality instead of being "good old Pat".'

Many of our members joined Pat in this last remark — they said that being thin meant that for the first time they could afford to have their own opinions rather than agreeing with everyone else so that people would like to have them around.

One of the most heart-warming stories concerned a husband and wife who were both Weight Watchers members. Peter was 7 stone overweight, a printer working for a major Sunday newspaper. His baby son had suffered brain damage as a result of 'cot disease injury'. One night Peter came home from work and stood by the cot looking down at his son. He suddenly realised that here was a child who would need him for the rest of his life — yet the way Peter was living, he might not be around for long. He joined Weight Watchers and lost weight rapidly. Later he brought his wife along too. She was overweight, and because of this and the stress of coping with their first child she was not anxious to have any more children. Losing weight gave her renewed confidence in herself and in their marriage; we were all thrilled to celebrate the birth of their second child.

Losing weight can have its amusing side too. From being a shy, retiring, self-conscious fatty, Birmingham member Vivienne Russell shed 73½ pounds of surplus fat to reduce her 16st 1½lb (102 kilo)figure to a trim 10st 12lb (65 kilos). Vivienne was no longer recognized when delivering work to a firm where she occasionally helped out. 'What's happened to that big fat woman who used to work at home for us?' asked a secretary. 'Isn't she working for us any more?' 'No,' said Vivienne with a smile, 'she's disappeared — and she won't be back!'

Then there was Madge Parnell who was so fat that every time she turned over in bed her husband Bill would roll towards her. The only way he could get a good night's sleep was by insisting on single beds. When Madge joined Weight Watchers and slimmed down from nearly 19 stone (121 kilo) to 9st 11lb (63 kilos), it was he who suggested they go shopping for a new double bed.

Maurice Braines, from Enfield in North London, weighed more than 21 stone (134 kilo) on his wedding day. He tried everything: counting calories, intravenous injections at St Bartholomew's Hospital, and even a crash diet consisting only of three cups of tea and a few vitamin tablets a day. But along came Christmas and during a week of festivities, he ate and drank his way back up to 21 stone. When he joined Weight Watchers he learned our most important principle: if you are going to maintain your weight loss you must start to eat the way you intend to eat for the rest of your life. Maurice lost nearly 8 stone to become the darling of the Golders Green class; the women flattered him and noticed each new change of clothing — so much so that his wife began to come to class to chaperone him!

The story of member Edna Plante was truly inspirational. One clear July afternoon, Edna crested the 4,406-foot Ben Nevis and gave a whoop of joy. After four hours' strenuous exertion she had climbed Britain's highest mountain, with energy to spare. Yet only three years earlier she couldn't climb the stairs without feeling breathless. Then 15 st 4 lb (98 kilos) she suffered palpitations of the heart, and at 43 seemed set for a premature old age — until she took the first step on her personal mountain and joined the local Weight Watchers class in Barnes. In eight months she trimmed off 81 pounds of excess fat, felt ten years younger and took up an exercise programme which eventually led to her mountain-climbing feat.

For 30-year-old Newton Abbot shop-owner Mark Charman, the turning point in a life of compulsive eating came after Christmas 1973 when he burst the seams of his 46-inch waist trousers. Ashamed and miserable, a history of failed dieting behind him and well aware of the health risk — Mark's mother died when he was 12 from an illness aggravated by overeating — he went with a friend to Weight Watchers. More than 84 pounds lighter at 12 st 12 lb (83 kilos), Mark's business had doubled, he was able to join in his small daughters' games for the first time, and he and his wife had taken up tennis, swimming and badminton.

'At school, I was always the boy on the touchline,' said Mark. 'Nowadays I'm so busy doing there's no time for looking on.'

Susan Thompson was another success story. At 21 she was 5 feet 2 inches tall but weighed 12½ stone (80 kilos); her roly-poly figure caused her to become too shy to visit friends or even leave her home near Dover to go out shopping. On the day she was 25 Susan woke up to the fact that life was passing her by and she suddenly became very angry with herself.

After joining Weight Watchers she turned into a stunning young woman with near-perfect measurements of 35–24–35, tipping the scales at 7st 8lb (50 kilos). She transformed herself from the 'Wide Hips of Dover' to be crowned Miss Dover two years running.

Margaret Smith of the Battersea class lost 98 pounds to change from a 54–44–56 figure to a trim 37–29–38. While she was attending Weight Watchers, her son was in Switzerland. He returned unexpectedly months later, looked at the strange woman in his home and asked: 'Where's Mum?' Only when he took a second, closer look did he realize that this *was* his mum.

Joining Weight Watchers also helped so many to fulfil their dreams. Sixteen-year-old Douglas Bray had a burning ambition to join the Army but was turned down because he was too fat. His mother tried him on various diets but nothing worked. In despair he joined the Plymouth Weight Watchers class, lost 2 stone (13 kilo) and regained his confidence. The Army then welcomed him second time round.

Mavis Holden wanted to emigrate to Australia with her husband Alf. Their application was turned down because the authorities thought Mavis (at 19 stone, 121 kilos) was so fat the journey might kill her. Weight Watchers came to the rescue. Just a year later Mavis was flying out to Sydney, New South Wales, and a new life in a new continent.

Other stories were more poignant. Margaret Cowling's weight problems nearly ruined her life. When she married, aged 18, she was slim; 25 years later her weight soared to 18 stone (115 kilos). She became a prisoner of her own body, staying in bed most of the day, getting up only in the afternoon to do housework. A special pulley had to be put up over her bed so that she could heave herself into a sitting position. She never ate with her family and wouldn't go near a window in case anyone outside saw her. The more reclusive she became, the bossier her behaviour was. She ruled her family with a rod of iron. When her children were married she didn't even go to their weddings. One day one of her sons lost his temper and accused her of looking — and behaving — like King Kong. A startled Margaret dragged herself to the mirror and finally faced what she had become. That was the turning point. She became a member of Weight Watchers and successfully reached her goal weight of 9 stone (57 kilos). But the nicest thing happened 'on the way to goal'. When I awarded her her 100-pound Loser's Certificate at a special ceremony, her family presented her with a beautiful gold watch; they had each invested £1 for every pound in weight she had lost in order to give her this special treat. She was overwhelmed by all the time and thought they too had invested in her success. This story helped also to illustrate to fellow members the wider role of Weight Watchers within the entire family — Margaret lost weight and all the Cowlings benefitted from that loss, becoming a happy and united family once again. Family members could be very supportive. I suggested that members enlist the aid and encouragement of their children. Some of the children even acted as 'vigilantes', turning their mothers in when they cheated.

One example of the way a child responded to this invitation involved Doreen Rigby. Her teenage son was on the verge of leaving school and going to university. When his mother reached goal weight and received her Weight Watchers pin she read out part of an essay written by her son. It was entitled 'The Most Important Event of 1968' and it began, 'The most important and exhilarating event I have experienced in 1968, the year of Rhodesian UDI, was my mother's struggle to lose weight.' He went on to describe her progress with Weight Watchers and the pride he felt in seeing his mother succeed. This success and support encouraged the once-lonely Doreen to go on and become a lecturer, a supervisor and eventually a regional manager, whom we turned to whenever we needed a self-confident representative.

Losing weight seemed to create new energy in people. Married couples claimed that they found it possible to use this energy to revitalize their marriages.

There were cases where people who lost huge amounts of weight suddenly discovered not only new energy and new self-confidence but a new sexuality. Often this improved the quality of their marriage — husbands frequently taking a greater interest in their wives and wives responding to this new ardour. They claimed a loss of weight improved their marriage by 'bringing them closer together'.

Thus when a journalist from the tabloid press tried to suggest that Weight Watchers was somehow responsible in some way for 'wrecking marriages', I was ready to do battle to refute the charge.

The journalist in question came to cover our first Weight Watchers holiday which we held in Harrogate. In 1973 Lord Forte, always a forward-thinking and imaginative entrepreneur, realized that people on diets frequently avoided holidays in hotels. He allowed us to experiment with the first ever diet holiday in Britain and gave us every assistance with staff and facilities. Members attending ranged from 8 stone (51 kilos) for the lightest lady to 28 st 3 lb (148 kilos). The idea proved a tremendous success — at the end of the week the 77 members attending had lost 25 stone (159 kilos) between them. But it came close to being marred by this journalist who, instead of reporting the event as news, spent his time prying and encouraging the women to talk about their 'love lives'. He was so charming that a few of our members actually made up stories just to catch his interest.

By coincidence one of the printers at the newspaper was a member of Weight Watchers. When he saw the story being set up in type he alerted me. I took legal advice immediately. It would have been possible to obtain an injunction to prevent the story from being used — it just wasn't true — but I was warned that legal action would create even more publicity of the kind that would upset both our members and their partners. Instead I arranged to meet a top executive from the paper.

He invited me to have a drink with him at a Fleet Street pub and suggested that he would be happy to 'kill' the story if I gave him some dirt on my relationship with Richard. He seemed to find it hard to believe that I hadn't had a series of affairs, and was disappointed when I told him that my husband was the only man in my life. I suggested that he report, instead, that in my efforts to stop my husband's night-eating syndrome, I would wear a small sign on my nightdress which read 'Reach for your Mate instead of your Plate'.

Despite incidents such as these, success bred success. Every transformation, every case history reported, proved a spur to others. Different people responded in different ways. Some enjoyed the competitiveness; they wanted to be the class champion. Others felt they couldn't let the group down. It didn't matter what the catalyst was — they all seemed to find their own way to successful weight loss.

The average weight loss was about 2—2½ pounds per week. Heavier people tended to lose weight more quickly. I remember in our Kingston class when Viv Davis returned to class after only one week on the Programme — the scales registered a 1 stone loss. I made her get off, checked the scales and she got on again. The scales still read the same. Laura Dance, my clerk, turned the scales completely upside down to see if anything was amiss, and finally we called a maintenance engineer. The scales were accurate; Viv had lost a whole stone. Later she became a lecturer and dazzled members with her story, though she was always the first to point out to them that in fact it was not the *amount* lost that was significant so much as successfully sticking to the Programme for another week. If a member had faith-fully done so then any amount lost, even half a pound, was a significant victory.

Sometimes members would complain that they weren't losing weight fast enough and we would point out that speed wasn't the object of the Weight Watchers Programme; the aim was to teach members how to eat properly, to find a new healthy weight for themselves and most importantly to learn how to maintain that weight.

Of course, not everyone who joined Weight Watchers stayed the course. About five per cent dropped out after one meeting. We always insisted that people who had a medical problem returned with a note from their doctor saying that it was all right for them to go on the Programme; some of these people were among the early drop-outs, perhaps because they didn't want to 'bother' their GPs. Then there were those who thought the Programme was too stringent or who had simply come along for yet another diet and were not prepared to make the commitment of coming every week. We didn't mind losing those — we didn't want casual slimmers.

Of those who got beyond the early stage, almost ninety-three per cent went on to reach and maintain their goal weight. Those who didn't tended to be people who had failed to follow the diet. They were 'expert' dieters who thought they could take any diet and change it to suit themselves. That change invited disaster.

There were some people who lost 3—5 stones (around 25 kilos) and decided to continue on their own, or else they felt that the goal we gave them was unrealistic and they were happy losing a smaller amount of weight. Research showed that people who left class before reaching goal never got there on their own. They also tended to regain the weight they had lost very quickly.

To reward people for staying the course and for losing weight we had a system of awarding Weight Watchers pins with diamante chips. Members were given this award after attending class for a minimum of 16 weeks and having lost a minimum of 10 pounds. After that, an extra chip was added for every additional 10 pounds you lost.

If you attended classes for a minimum of 16 weeks and reached goal weight, you were given free lifetime member-ship. You no longer had to pay for classes, provided you came once a month. If, however, your weight was more than 22 pounds over goal you had to pay the normal weekly fee. The same applied if you missed a monthly meeting. The purpose here was to encourage members to stay active — like diabetics, we felt they needed a regular 'fix'.

Because I knew that Weight Watchers was often someone's last hope, I was always very concerned about 'drop-out-ism'. In the early days it was possible for me to keep track of the progress of almost every member in every class, but as the organization grew I set up new follow-up methods. I insisted that lecturers ring up members who missed a class, or whose weight loss appeared irregular. Those who didn't contribute to group discussions were often sought out privately by friendly telephone calls. All of this added to the costs of running Weight Watchers since we reimbursed the lecturers for their time and the cost of their call, but I felt all this was essential.

We discovered that 'drop-out-ism' was something that affected fat people generally. They started project after project, lost heart or didn't have the energy, and gave up. This was true of some who joined Weight Watchers. It was a problem that particularly interested me and when I discovered a new course called 'synectics', I subjected myself, members of our head office staff, lecturers and supervisors to a guinea pig course. We were all so elated by our success with this new method of teaching and strengthening resolve that we decided to bring it to the classes. Synectics was frequently called 'the art of positive thinking'. In reality it trained people's thinking in such a way as to reduce the scale of the problem they faced or conversely in some instances to exaggerate the scope so that the problem was more clearly evident, as was the solution.

When, in my weekly meetings with supervisors, I discovered that there was a large drop-out problem in the Slough class I decided to try out synectics there. While the lecturer ran the class in the front of the room, I took those with the most irregular attendance record to the back. We chose one woman and asked her what her greatest problem was. She explained that her husband worked nights, that she was frequently left on her own and found it difficult not to binge in the evenings to make up for her loneliness.

We decided to break down the various parts of that problem and listed on a blackboard all the different possibilities which we called 'how to's': each member of the group made a suggestion and by the end of that round we had 'how to's' such as how to keep one's hands busy with things other than eating, how to find ways to make the evenings constructive, how to pursue night courses, and how to find a lover.

The group pounced on this last possibility and in our discussion it became obvious that one of the answers was to lose weight and become more attractive.

During the course of that meeting I discovered that this inner group had formed a clique of ladies who left the class each week and celebrated in a nearby pub. Most of them broke their diet as soon as that happened. I suggested that they use the visit to the pub this time to scout out a 'potential lover'.

The group apparently piled out to help the woman make her selection. They were all so fascinated by her project that they kept phoning round all week, thereby encouraging one another to stick to the diet. Next week they all came back and with them brought others who had dropped out on other occasions. The class involvement was astonishing. The results were heartening. The member in question lost so much weight and became so attractive that her husband took a far greater interest in her. In the evenings she began studying sociology, psychology and even began reading sex manuals. Her husband, at first alarmed, became interested too in her reading selections and before long they were experimenting happily together. He chose a new job working in the day time!

It became clear that if you followed the Programme you were virtually 100 per cent certain of losing weight in a healthy natural way. Even those who had failed consistently on other diets found Weight Watchers remarkably effective.

Dolly Wager proved this point dramatically. Like so many other fat people her weight problems had created a spiral of depression and overeating. The fatter she became, the more depressed she felt — and therefore the more she ate. Doctor after doctor had washed his hands of her problem until a surgeon recommended a partial lobotomy, saying that she would never lose weight but at least surgery would minimize her depression.

Dolly joined Weight Watchers and went on to lose 20 stones (127 kilos)in 20 months. When she came to us, she weighed 31 st 2lb (199 kilos) and measured 76–75–78. She would eat an entire loaf of bread, cut into sandwiches, for tea alone. With Weight Watchers' help, she changed from what she described as a 'thing' into a trim forty-year-old attractive woman weighing 11 stone (70 kilo)and measuring 36–28–37. Her husband Dave was in ecstasy and thoroughly spoiled the new Dolly.

They both went to America to represent British Weight Watchers at the New York Weight Watchers' birthday celebrations. When Dolly left from Heathrow, one of our members, the Manager of Billy Smart's Circus and Safari Park in Windsor, brought along a small elephant to weigh on the scale with Dolly. All Weight Watchers in Great Britain signed a huge birthday card which we gave Dolly to take to Jean Nidetch. As I watched her walk to the plane with Dave, I knew that miracles do happen — but these were miracles that we made with our own hands.

Dolly's story was out of the ordinary in many ways, yet at the same time she was the perfect illustration of the magic of Weight Watchers. The magic lay in seeing people who came in, imprisoned in their own fat, and watching the Programme work for them. They would tell stories of how they had tried everything — and failed. Then, week by week, you would see chinks appearing in their terrible prison until out came the most beautiful women, like butterflies from a chrysalis.

CHAPTER SIX

As Dolly Wager realized, and every other person who has ever been fat knows, you don't put on weight overnight. Except in the most unusual circumstances, weight is put on over many months, or, more likely, over several years. Nor is losing weight simply a question of summoning up enough willpower to stick to a diet — whatever those who have never been fat may think! In fact, diets tend to have a built-in 'failure factor' for fat people — and most fat people simply do not have willpower. What a fat person can develop is discipline and sensible eating habits to substitute for that elusive willpower.

Weight Watchers, over the years, helped many millions of people to develop and maintain a regime — a way of life — which enabled them first to lose weight by eating sensibly and then to continue with that way of life, thus maintaining this weight loss. As a result, Weight Watchers became many things to many people — it was often not considered a business at all.

In the earliest days, church and school officials offered us their meeting halls free of charge, seeing us as a non-profit-making organization; we told them that that was not what we had intended — it just seemed that way at the beginning. Later, when 500 lecturers were depositing their daily or evening receipts in their local branches of Barclays Bank, the bank's chairman told me we were not a weight loss business but in banking — and seriously so.

Others claimed we were adjuncts or allies to the medical and psychological professions, whilst a priest went so far as to claim our lecturers inspired people to confess more readily than he. We were even referred to by politicians as a 'pressure group'. Laura Dance, one of our ablest lecturers, advised us to 'sit on them' until they did what we wanted, claiming our 'pressure' would be weighty and effective.

We actually did become a very effective pressure group indeed, dealing with large and small issues. One of the larger issues was 'health education'.

When the British medical and scientific establishment finally started treated obesity with the seriousness it deserves, it worked unceasingly to spread the gospel. The leading lights in nutrition, metabolism and endocrinology combined with physicians who treated diabetes, high blood pressure, heart disease, arthritis, asthma, and other obesity-aggravated diseases.

The British Obesity Association was formed in 1970 under its first Chairman, Professor John Butterfield, now Lord Butterfield: a distinguished scientist, physician, hospital administrator and educator. He was a tireless campaigner for the promotion of health education. John Butterfield inspired his colleagues to treat this malady seriously and imaginatively. He was, and remains, indefatigable: no lecture, conference, seminar or congress too small or insignificant for his attention; and he graciously made those of us in Weight Watchers without professional qualifications (who were heretofore overwhelmed and underappreciated) feel that our contributions too were valuable. He inspired us to work even more closely with his medical and scientific colleagues, and entreated them to respect our contributions and reward our success. He was one of Weight Watchers' earliest and most enthusiastic supporters. As Vice-Chancellor of Cambridge University he raised public perception of the role of sport and fitness in maintaining health to new heights. Now, as Chairman of the Health Promotion Research Trust, he continues those efforts.

Our activities as a lay organization extended across a

broad spectrum. In conjunction with the British Heart Foundation we raised substantial sums through sponsored slimming events and other promotions such as 'Protect the Heart of the Man You Love'. We asked top London restaurants (as well as local bistros around the country) to serve Weight Watchers lunches to business executives. *Harpers* magazine ran a special feature reprinting the menus of hotels like the Savoy, the Ritz, Claridges, Grosvenor House and the Connaught, just to prove that expensive restaurant menus offered a wide choice of healthy non-fattening meals.

I returned to Harrods to wipe out the memory of my first defeat by this time convincing the restaurant to start serving Weight Watchers lunches and Weight Watchers teas for our members and for other patrons.

After I had written a second cook book, we used the launch of my third book, *Weight Watchers, A Way of Life* to raise money for the British Health Foundation and the Health Education Council, which was just being formed. We held the launch of the book on Valentine's Day and I presented a huge Weight Watchers valentine to our then overweight Prime Minister at No. 10 Downing Street. The Liberal MP Cyril Smith, never one to be taken lightly, graciously accepted a valentine as well.

In similar vein the Mayor of Windsor, Kit Aston, was warned by his physician to lose weight urgently. We turned his individual battle into a campaign to encourage other mayors and their council members throughout Great Britain to lose weight. They raised money for their favourite charities (as well as the Heart Foundation and Prince Philip's Silver Jubilee Fund) by encouraging people in their constituencies to sponsor them, 'a penny a pound'. The most successful mayor was in fact a mayoress: she rewarded me by allowing me to wear her chain of office for one evening.

Early on we began to reward those who had lost 50 pounds and others who had lost 100. In addition to their normal Weight Watchers graduation pin we wanted to honour these large losers, and by publicizing their success encourage people with comparable amounts to lose, to believe that the battle was worth fighting. Again, Lord Forte came to our aid by volunteering the use of his private apartment at the Café Royal for a special 50-pound loser class for men only. It was better than any stag party!

Men who wanted to lose 50 pounds met men who had already lost as much. The men-only format was thought to be best as there are some problems associated with obesity in men — urinary incompetence, for instance, which it might have been difficult to discuss in a mixed meeting.

Also at the Café Royal we had our first dinner dance for Weight Watchers lecturers and their husbands and wives. The catering manager told me later that he had never attended such a happy event. Every couple danced every dance and the mood was high, even though no alcohol was served.

Later we commenced exotic Weight Watchers holidays to the island of Elba in Italy, and to Spain, as well as other holidays in Britain. I remember a photograph sent to me of Molly West aged 66 dressed as a Hawaiian Hula dancer, entertaining both Weight Watchers and the local islanders. They applauded not only her dancing but her extraordinary figure which showed not a bulge remaining. Molly was a legend in our time. As a lecturer she woke early on market day to buy huge amounts of fish for those members of her class, who, as young mothers, were unable to get out to do proper Weight Watchers shopping. It thrills me that that extra burst of self-confidence which came to her with her weight reduction has not been lost even now. At 81 she visited me not long ago and when I commented on her extraordinary energy and physical vivacity, she said, 'And my mind and spirit are just as active. You know, I still have orgasms.'

In 1974 we launched a competition jointly with *TV Times* to find the Weight Watcher of the Year. It was one of our

most successful promotions. The deserving winner was
Jennifer Pincombe, a member of the Paignton class.
Jennifer had originally joined Weight Watchers some years
previously, after her doctor advised her to lose weight in
order to increase her chances of having the baby she so
desperately wanted.

Jennifer lost weight — and went on to have four children
— but failed to stick to the maintenance programme and
soon found the pounds piling back on. When she rejoined
Weight Watchers she was 17st 13lb (115 kilos), and looked
more like a grandmother of 58 than a mother of 28. Slowly
but surely the weight came off again until she was back at a
trim 10st (64 kilo) with a figure that measured 36–30–38
rather than 46–39½–52. The transformation was dramatic:
when you looked at her before and after photographs it was
almost impossible to believe it was the same woman.

We began a series of behaviour modification training
programmes for our lecturers in association with the Institute of Behaviour Modification in London. Closed circuit
television filmed the effects of these behavioural techniques
on weight and weight-related problems. These films were
later used as excellent teaching devices, not only for our
members and staff, but for use in hospital behavioural
programmes and by schools and local health centres.

We sponsored the first medical seminar on obesity at
which Professor Henry J. Sebrell spoke at the Royal Society
and the Royal Society of Medicine. Professor Sebrell had
been the Assistant Director of the National Institute of
Health in Washington and much impressed the British
physicians who attended with his pragmatic approach and
deep sympathy for the overweight. He stressed how helpful
behaviour therapy had been in identifying the peculiar
needs and attitudes of his obese patients. In one of his
famous experiments, obese medical students and normal
students were asked to 'suck out' of a feeding machine all
their daily dietary and nutritional requirements. The
normal students satisfied their usual calorie needs, but the

fat students, to whom eating was a sensual and exotic experience, ate not at all from this uninteresting machine. Hooray — at least a few points for the sensibility of the obese who were otherwise considered almost loutish in their approach to food.

This seminar was followed by the first ever Psychological Conference on Obesity, which introduced Professor Stanley Schachter of the Columbia University Institute for Human Nutrition to the British public. He was a marvellously funny man and a scientist par excellence. Unfortunately his excessive consumption of cigarettes during the meeting caused one British physician to say: 'I'll give up chocolates if you give up smoking.' Professor Schachter encouraged us to study the effect that external cues have in triggering the obese to eat. We discovered to our amazement that in a controlled experiment, the group that was over-fed (uncomfortably so) was more likely to buy large amounts in a supermarket (with the same amount of money) than those who had been without food for a longer period and who were quite peckish. In essence we discovered that the act of eating is itself a stimulant to the fat person. Weight Watchers received much acclaim for bringing this extraordinary scientist to Britain.

Although the term behaviour modification is used today on a grand scale and describes many projects and activities now used by slimming organizations (government sponsored and private), it was first popularized through the publication of Dr Richard Stuart's small volume *A Slim Chance in a Fat World*. Later we brought Professor Stuart (who had become a psychological adviser to Weight Watchers International) to Britain where he created quite a stir in English and Scottish medical circles. My lecturers and I used his modules in this country and adapted them for indigenous British use. Some of his inspired theories have become perhaps the most successful and widely accepted formulae for the treatment of obesity in this country.

My lecturers and I experimented with these concepts and with the modules devised by Dr Stuart in his approach to the treatment of obesity through behaviour modification. We found from our experience that these techniques added magically to our success and I would like to share with you some of the major tools we used and the rules by which we learned successfully to maintain our weight loss.

1. **NEVER, NEVER COUNT CALORIES OR CARBOHYDRATE UNITS.** It positively encourages you to eat the wrong food and skip the essentials you need for a balanced diet. It may even encourage you to eat extra large meals and skip others to even out the count.

2. **EAT BETWEEN MEALS.** If you are a nibbler and get hungry between meals don't suffer hunger pains — nibble — or else you will eat in an unbalanced way. Make yourself a Weight Watcher popcorn bowl or a cucumber, watercress and pimento salad, or freshly grilled mushrooms. (Don't crash diet, it's unhealthy.)

3. **DON'T SKIP MEALS.** A missed meal doesn't mean a slimmer you, it upsets the balance of your eating pattern and encourages you to eat extra large meals afterwards. Also, meal eaters burn off ten per cent more calories than meal skippers because every time they eat their metabolic rate goes up.

4. **DON'T WEIGH YOURSELF CONSTANTLY WHILE LOSING WEIGHT.** Once a week is quite enough.

5. **DON'T GO INTO COMPETITION WITH ANOTHER DIETER.** No two people lose weight at the same rate (not even identical twins).

6. **EAT BEFORE YOU GO TO A PARTY.** If you arrive quite full and aren't hungry you won't be tempted to eat the

canapés and dips and other goodies you shouldn't. You might even eat a complete meal at home before going to the party ... or else eat afterwards.

7. **DON'T SHUT YOURSELF AWAY WHILST SLIMMING.** Lead your normal life — otherwise you will only think slim when you are in a shut-away environment and sensible eating will collapse when you return to your normal routine.

8. **REMEMBER, OTHER PEOPLE MAY NOT WANT YOU TO SUCCEED.** Friends and family may 'like to see you as you are'.

9. **DON'T TALK ABOUT YOUR SLIMMING REGIME TO OTHER PEOPLE.** Save your conversation for your class or for friends on a similar regime.

10. **NEVER SAY 'DIET'. THE BEST LOSERS CHANGE THEIR WAY OF EATING FOR LIFE.** Going on a diet also implies going off a diet.

11. **BE REALISTIC — TRYING TO SHRINK TO AN IMPOSSIBLY LOW WEIGHT DOOMS YOU TO DEFEAT.** Rapid loss diets are ultimately damaging both physically and psychologically.

12. **COMMON PITFALLS OF ALL LOW-CALORIE DIETS ARE THE LACK OF ADEQUATE BEHAVIOUR MODIFICATION AND FOLLOW-UP.** When you stop the diet and put the pounds back on you feel like a failure and studies show that next time you try to lose weight it will take longer and you will gain even more weight back. Therefore the wiser course is start slowly and make steady progress, peel off 1 to 2 pounds a week.

13. **MAKE ONE CHANGE AT A TIME.** Too much deprivation can leave you ripe for a binge.

14. **KEEP A DIET DIARY — RECORD EVERY MORSEL THAT GOES INTO YOUR MOUTH**. Read your diary frequently to find out more about what, when and where you eat and why.

To stop people cheating we used to get them to write little poems about it. We gave them stickers to put on their fridges saying things like: 'Who are you angry with?' because when you are angry with someone the first thing you do is go straight to the fridge. To stop people eating in the night we suggested they should reach for their mate, not their plate, and we had another sticker which read: 'Make love, not midnight snacks'.

We encouraged people to keep diaries so that they could identify when they were most likely to cheat. By recognizing their weak moments they could plan ahead in order to avoid temptation in the first place. For example, we found that woman who went out to work often cheated when it was time for elevenses. Round came the tea trolley with drinks, biscuits and buns and it was hard for them to resist.

Housewives often hit a low at the same time of the morning. Having started the day with good intentions about getting all the chores done before lunchtime, they would suddenly be struck with a bout of 'can't-cope-itis' at around eleven o'clock when they realized the morning was half over and the house still looked as if a bomb had hit it. To cheer themselves up they sat down with a cup of coffee, a magazine — and something to eat. Our advice was to remove yourself from temptation: go to the ladies' when the trolley came round, or get out of the house mid-morning. Another tactic was to make sure that there was nothing around that would tempt you to cheat. We always told members that cheating began in the supermarket: that was where you bought the foods that caused your downfall. So we advised people never to shop when they were hungry, and to make a list — and stick to it. We also told them that there was no reason why their families should not eat the same foods as they did. You didn't have to buy sweets and chocolates for everyone else and then feel you were missing out on something.

One of the best things about Weight Watchers was that we accepted that our members would eat between meals so the Programme included 'legal' snacks. One suggestion I used to make was that people should take time to make up a whole bowl of what we called number three vegetables — the ones you could eat either in unlimited quantities or in moderate amounts every day. The idea was to wash them, slice them up and keep them in an enormous bowl in the fridge with a label on it saying 'Eat me'. When you opened the door, that would be the first thing you saw.

If people didn't lose weight on the Programme, we would be pretty sure they were cheating, but getting them to admit it wasn't always easy. Betty Clark, one of the early members, really had me puzzled. Her weight was constantly going up and down, yet she swore she wasn't cheating at all. Finally I rang her one evening from a hotel 200 miles away and quizzed her again. Only then, at a safe distance from me, could she admit the truth: she was.

Of course, there were inevitably times when temptation in one form or another simply proved too much for people — but we used to warn our members that there was a good chance their sins would find them out. Remember the doughnut episode if ever you are tempted!

You will find at the back of this book an Appendix in which are some of my favourite recipes. You will learn quickly that they are very 'heavy' on dessert — I *love* desserts — but also included are some of my recommended recipes for soups, entrées, sauces, dressings, for salads and vegetables and other staples, which I have enjoyed over the years and still enjoy to this day.

Whenever I found myself at a loss I picked myself up with a tasty — but, even more important, attractive-looking — starter such as Baked Apples Stuffed with Raspberries. I also used it as a dessert because it impressed my dinner guests with its texture, colour, taste and aroma.

At elevenses I would have a mid-morning bouillon or a 'legal' milkshake or a Golden Grapefruit.

My soups were a lifesaver. I always had large jars of prepared diet soups ready in the fridge or in the freezer for the times when I raced into the house late and hungry. Sipping soup took the edge off my hunger — and prevented me from tearing into a packet and getting myself in trouble. I'm a chocoholic but even I have to admit it doesn't taste so good after a perfectly 'legal' shake of crunchy grilled mushrooms spiked with garlic salt.

I loved serving Yorkshire Pudding or Shepherd's Pie, Weight Watchers-style, and causing my guests to wonder how these dishes could be slimming. I further amazed them with desserts such as crumbles, soufflés and sorbets.

And, of course, for special occasions when I wanted to knock everyone's eyes out there was Chocolate Cake Bérénice. It was a tour de force — and no one would believe it was not terribly fattening. (It could be — if you ate it all at once and by yourself!)

Do try my favourites included in the Appendix — but do eat them slowly, savour each bite as you would any sensual experience. And ENJOY!

CHAPTER SEVEN

We decided to celebrate Weight Watchers' fifth birthday in style. By holding a special event to mark the occasion we could not only look back at everything which had happened in the years between 1967 and 1972, but look forward to all the exciting plans we had for the future.

My first idea was to hold a rally in Hyde Park but Richard pointed out that the British weather could all too easily put a damper on such an event. Instead we decided to hold a whale of a party in the Royal Albert Hall. We had come a long way from the village hall in Datchet.

On January 8th 1972, traffic all around the Albert Hall ground to a halt as thousands of our members arrived in coaches, cars and taxis from all parts of the country. There was only room for 6,000 so we held a draw for places, and were sorry to disappoint the thousands more who were unlucky. Even so, hundreds turned up on the off-chance that they might be able to take part.

The stage was built to look like a giant birthday cake and an enormous golden weighing-in scale towered over it. Richard masterminded the design and was on his best form as Master of Ceremonies. The whole evening was electrifying. Calypso singer Cy Grant wrote and performed a special Weight Watchers calypso for the occasion and everyone joined in the chorus. World weight-lifting champion Louis Martin presided over the special weigh-in for six of our top losers who now each weighed less than the amount of weight they had lost.

All the key people were there: the first members, the first

lecturers, even the man who threw us out of his pub when he learned that Weight Watchers banned alcohol.

Miriam Karlin told the story of how she was turned away by Weight Watchers. Roald Dahl and his wife Patricia Neal were our special guests who accepted a Weight Watchers cheque to be donated to the NSPCC.

My children still remember sitting in a box with their nanny, watching spellbound, and I'm not surprised. It was a fairy-tale occasion and at the end, amidst the popping of diet drink cans (with a stray bottle of champagne), and balloons and streamers drifting down from the balcony, everyone linked arms and sang. The atmosphere was as emotional as a revival meeting and everyone was uplifted by the sheer joy of it all, the joy that Weight Watchers had brought to so many people.

Yet it was ironic that despite our success — in fact, because of it — Weight Watchers was beginning to bring me anything but joy.

Everything had been marvellous while Richard and I could control things down to the very last detail; when we had a limited number of lecturers each of whom ran two or three classes. But now we were growing so fast that we needed more people to help with administration: we were fast becoming a national organization. Weight Watchers in America was a series of smaller franchises: no one else had a franchise covering 52 million people, as we did, so there was no advice the Americans could give us; there were no guidelines to follow. Once again, it was up to us to find our own way to make things work.

We had long since moved from our office above the betting shop in Datchet into charming, spacious offices in Windsor, overlooking the Castle, and we had been lucky in our appointment of Leslie Levonton as general manager. Neither Richard nor I knew how to set up a national organization and administer it, whereas Leslie was experienced in setting up retail fashion outlets for national clothing chains. He was accustomed to working with large

numbers of women whom he inspired by making them feel
valued and special. This was of key importance to us since
most of our lecturers were women. Actually, during the first
ten years of Weight Watchers in the UK there were only, at
the very most, five male lecturers. This was because people
seemed to respond better to the mother figure and also
because at the very beginning, lecturing for Weight
Watchers was only a part-time job. Although it was possible
to earn reasonable money, it didn't pay enough for a man
to support his family.

There weren't many men who were able to run a class in
the evening after a day at their own job, although to be fair
there were many who came to help their lecturer wives,
acting as clerks or weighers, or just by setting up the chairs
and props for the meetings.

Although I had a great deal of respect and admiration for
Leslie, as time went on I found myself disagreeing with
him. He wanted to keep the status quo, to keep things
simple, whereas I wanted to refine and improve the work
we were doing, to stimulate and inspire my lecturers for the
benefit of all members. Leslie often felt my innovations
were not cost-effective. No one could have been more
skilled at the difficult task of keeping everything running
smoothly but, as a businessman, Leslie loved the mechanics
of business, the patterns of expansion and growth.

As we grew, we had to bring in other professionals, such
as financial advisers, and all too often Leslie, Richard and
'the others', as I thought of them, were in total agreement
and I was outvoted more and more often.

Take the issue of advertizing, for instance. I always
believed that editorial coverage was worth far more than
advertizing. The press loved a good 'before and after' story
and were as keen to run them as we were to have them
printed. But during the time I was in hospital after having
our third child, Leslie and Richard hired a top advertizing
agency and paid for full-page advertizements in the *Daily
Express* and other newspapers. Not only did this effectively

discourage newspapers from running stories about us (the ad managers on the papers started to tell the editorial staff not to write about us unless we advertized as well) but, worst of all, the campaign itself turned out to be a total waste of money. It pulled in fewer than 16 new members and made Weight Watchers seem like just another slimming business, rather than a grass roots, almost evangelical movement.

I had felt since the beginning that advertizing would not attract the kinds of people who needed Weight Watchers. People who came to our classes had stopped believing in pills, diets and fads. They had tried everything like that in the past — and failed. A slick, smart ad was unlikely to draw them in.

So the advertizing campaign was not only counter-productive in terms of free publicity, I felt we had wasted money that I would have preferred to invest in training or underwriting research to extend our services.

Richard and Leslie believed in statistics and graphs and economic consultants. Like many men, Richard loved com-puters, print-outs and charts. My interests were exactly the opposite. Whereas I spent my time preparing lectures, reading reports from the classes and being 'in touch', he was reading only the financial reports. Richard used to say that when the computer heard my feet on the stairs it stopped working because it knew I didn't believe in it, and he was right, I didn't. I didn't need a chart. I could tell exactly how things were going merely from talking to our lecturers or supervisors in the field.

It seemed to me that the men were distancing themselves from the brave, wonderful, intelligent Weight Watchers members. This disturbed me deeply. I felt more and more alone: tolerated by uninvolved experts. I felt as if I had to fight not only to protect my personal integrity and my commitment to the ideals of Weight Watchers, but for recognition of and respect from every Weight Watchers member as a person rather than a statistic.

That's why the lecturers were so important, why they had to be chosen and supervised so carefully. Anyone coming to Weight Watchers was like a drowning man going down for the third time. We were their last chance: we just couldn't fail them. But the 'professionals' were taking away the human touch. They began sending out lecturers before they were totally prepared. It was just a numbers game to them and it upset me when I thought about the time and trouble I had taken in the past.

One woman, for instance, who really deserved to be a lecturer had failed twice to meet the standards and quality. I felt she had the ability and very special qualities but that her failure was due to nervousness.

The third time she was tested she travelled all the way from Coventry to our home at Datchet, and her whole family came with her to give her support. I tried to make her as comfortable as possible. My sons were ready for bed but they came in in their pyjamas and performed a little song-and-dance act, and by the time she took her test and showed me what she could do, she was relaxed and confident. Her basic sincerity and strength came through as I had hoped — and she passed. I was so thrilled that I kissed her. Later I was told that this kind of behaviour was inappropriate, that our organization was too large and I was too important for that kind of display.

I felt the criticism was harsh and ran counter to the free and natural exchanges I enjoyed with the lecturers and members. I felt that all effort, all improvement, should be praised, shared and encouraged.

Our administrators' attitude to the lecturers was different from mine. I knew from my own experiences of trying to run classes while fitting in time with my children that it was important for a lecturer to be able to open a class in a place that suited her and her family, at a time which was convenient to them. But these men were now insisting that while our system might have been acceptable in the early days, it wasn't the way to run a sophisticated business.

Now, I was told, it was for our administrators to decide where the classes should be and it was up to the lecturer to follow orders. It didn't matter that she might end up arguing with her husband or having to leave her children before they were ready for bed. If someone wanted to work for us, they said, she would have to accept that this was the way things were run in the business world.

One of the rules I had instituted earlier was that if a member of the public joined a Weight Watchers class we wouldn't close that class around them. Since weighing in each week was so important, we would keep the class going — even if it meant running at a loss — until every member of that class found another Weight Watchers group.

Because of that policy it was risky to expand at breakneck speed unless you were certain that classes you were opening had a big enough catchment area and the demand was there. Again, our new administrators became so carried away with their graphs and their charts that they opened up 120 new classes in a very short space of time and as a result the break-even figure per class shot up radically. When they realized they couldn't simply close the more poorly attended classes (because I wouldn't let them), they decided they would balance the book-keeping figures by reducing the lecturers' pay.

The plan was to cut basic salaries and force lecturers to rely more on the commission that was paid according to the numbers in a class. When those in the field heard about this, they threatened to go on strike. Although the whole affair was dreamed up without my knowledge, I was the one Richard and Leslie asked to travel round the country from area to area to talk the women out of it.

I agreed to do this only if I could explain to the lecturers that it was all a mistake and that things would continue as before. Even this required a hard-fought battle on my part, Richard taking the position that bosses never apologized and didn't have to explain.

Time and time again I found myself at loggerheads with

the professionals Richard and Leslie had brought in over my refusal to compromise on issues I held dear. At one stage I remember being involved in a publicity campaign for my second cook book. I turned up as requested by the publisher's advertising agency in a studio to have some photographs taken, only to be confronted with a lifesize cardboard cut-out of a very fat headless woman. I was supposed to stand so that my head appeared on top of this gross body and have a photograph taken in order to suggest that this was one of my 'before' pictures.

When I refused to do it, none of the ad executives of the then fledgling Saatchi & Saatchi could understand why I was making such a fuss, but I knew my instincts were right. Apart from the fact that my genuine 'before' pictures were used in every class, Weight Watchers had been built up around authenticity and honesty. We had made 'before and after' pictures so famous that everyone trying to sell diets and slimming aids was now using them — and far too many of them showed fanciful 'before' pictures of a woman in a heavy jumper, slumped over, looking as fat as possible, while her 'after' pictures portrayed her standing up straight in a flimsy cotton dress. Fat people could spot those kind of tricks a mile off, and Weight Watchers respected the truth.

Another example of what happened when the professionals took over was the opening of Weight Watchers in Glasgow. A public relations firm was hired to organize our first open meeting. The event was to be televized with me addressing an audience of potential Weight Watchers. It was the first time I hadn't handled a promotion of this kind myself.

When I arrived to give my lecture I walked into a room in which there was not one woman under 60 and not one over 8 stone. All my fat jokes went right out of the window but I ploughed bravely on. At the end there was just one question.

A woman asked how much it cost to join. I told her it was £1 to register and 14 shillings a week. 'And do we get three meals a day for our 14 shillings?' she wanted to know. Now I knew I was in Scotland.

In spite of all my travelling during this period of rapid expansion, I was still enjoying family life.

We adored our new baby; she was strong, healthy and almost precocious: she walked at ten months and spoke remarkably well by one year, and I felt torn between the business and my children. The boys were inordinately energetic and talented, and whereas we both killed ourselves to be there at every sports event, play or other school function, there was no mistaking the fact that I was not there for them at all times which is an important thing for a child to know. In retrospect I feel as all working mothers feel or have felt — that I cheated myself and the children in terms of the time we might have spent together. Weight Watchers had become in a sense another child which had begun to demand a disproportionate share of my time, love and energies. Yet I know that my work with Weight Watchers changed the lives of hundreds of men and women, and created happier people, happier workmates, happier families.

However happiness in my own personal life remained elusive. Though Richard and I were united in our love for our children, there were constant undertows of stress within our marriage. Ironically, one of the chief of these was Richard's failure to accept rules, such as those of healthy eating. This worried me because he had gout and other medical complications which he refused to take seriously.

Although he had many wonderful qualities, Richard just didn't have a Weight Watchers mentality. That meant sticking at it, coming to class, being part of a group, giving and getting support. It meant accepting that there were no special rules for him, that there were individual commitments and commitments to the group and that our Programme of Eating was something which had to be followed exactly. Unfortunately Richard never really accepted the basic wisdom of Weight Watchers rules.

One particular incident stands out in my mind. One Sunday my sons and I wanted to visit London. Richard took us all to the Lyons Corner House at Marble Arch. He and I ordered perfectly 'legal' meals for ourselves and the children but, despite my wishes, Richard added an order of chips for the children. As soon as the food arrived he started sneaking chips off their plates. I became more and more distressed and pleaded with him. When the children's fruit dessert arrived, Richard ordered chocolate mousse for them 'as a treat'. He then pulled out the chocolate flakes and began to eat them. That was too much! I told him he was setting the children a bad example; he was far from goal and 'cheating' — and I was not staying to watch. I took all the left-over chips and the mousse and pushed the whole lot in front of him. Then I stormed out, leaving my handbag behind so that I was forced to hitch-hike all the way home to Datchet.

The incident had unforeseen consequences. The following Tuesday I had my weekly meeting with the lecturers, and Joyce Gourdie said very little: she had obviously encountered a problem in her class. Finally she admitted that one of her members had been in Lyons Corner House on Sunday and was now convinced that I didn't practise what I preached. She had witnessed me feeding my overweight husband chips and chocolate mousse! I told Joyce to go back and tell her lecturers to use that story, explaining what had happened and saying that the reason that attendance at Weight Watchers was important, because no wife was a good lecturer to her own husband, and vice versa. It was better for them to join a class and get motivated that way.

The Americans had originally set Richard's goal rather low. He did slim down from 19 (121 kilos) to 14½ stone (94 kilos) — a magnificent achievement. He looked marvellous and everyone noted and complimented him on how elegant he looked. To encourage him, I bought him new brightly coloured shirts and accessories from Turnbull & Asser and together we shopped for and ordered new suits. But fighting obesity is a persistent battle; Richard was unfortunately much better with short-term goals. He became bored easily and liked 'moving on to something else'. Perhaps if he had not been Chairman of Weight Watchers, his weight would not have been so painful an issue. His failure was damaging, not only to him but to many who admired him, and particularly to the members of our staff who looked up to him. He went through a phase of attending various classes, promising each lecturer that he would return. She would feel excited and special and anticipate the kudos of succeeding in getting Richard's weight down where others had failed. He may have hoped for a breakthrough himself, but one after another he abandoned the classes and hurt and disappointed the lecturers.

Richard was a classic example of the professional dieter. He still thought of diets as something you went on and fell off; he never really embraced the idea that the Weight Watchers Programme was a way of life. For instance, we had planned a long weekend in France. My idea was that I could prove to Richard and to members back in our classes that it was possible to have a wonderful, active holiday without gaining weight while sticking rigidly to the Programme.

For several days we picnicked or ate in simple restaurants where we were able to order 'legal' food. Then we moved on to a hotel in Honfleur renowned for its chef. I ordered all our food, making sure that the fish was grilled without oil and the vegetables served without butter. On the second evening, at Richard's elbow on the table next to ours was a huge bowl of chocolate mousse. Halfway through our first course Richard suddenly started to tell me where I could find the plane tickets home, as well as the number of his safety deposit box and the details of his life insurance policies. I couldn't think why he was explaining all this until he suddenly announced that he was going to commit suicide: he would plunge his head into that bowl of mousse and suffocate himself in chocolate.

Although Richard made light of it, what he was saying was serious indeed. He felt that life was hardly worth living if he was to be deprived of his favourite foods. And he had so many favourite foods ...

After that holiday (in which he did manage to lose 10 pounds), trying to stop him cheating became a losing battle. I would make sure he kept to the Programme at home but when he was out of sight, he would eat whatever he fancied and in large amounts. He seemed addicted to rich, exotic, gourmet food. When he first began to regain weight he made jokes about it. His humour and self-deprecation were beguiling at first, but later these jokes grew tiresome — particularly to those members of staff who accepted my ruling that any lecturer who was more than 5 pounds above her goal was obliged to suspend herself. Richard hated failing and was far too sensitive, too intelligent not to know how that failure upset me, and he knew it was trying to those members of our staff who lived Weight Watchers all the time proudly and publicly.

The situation became so painful that at 18 stone (115 kilos) again Richard began to avoid many of our public appearances, and to evade as many Weight Watchers contacts as possible. He no longer shared with me so many of the events that once had given us both so much joy, nor did he use his creative skills (which were far greater than mine) in creating public demonstrations of Weight Watchers' successes. This resulted in my having to carry a double load. I didn't understand, then, that Richard had begun to dislike Weight Watchers, and that this dislike would turn into an extreme jealously and hatred. Eventually he was determined, somehow or other, to separate us both from Weight Watchers if he could.

After our quarrels — loud, angry, hurtful exchanges — he had a formula for wordless repentance. First we made love in passionate reconciliation. Then I was wooed with flowers, expensive gifts, designer clothes — everything his extravagant and original mind could devise.

Gable House in Wentworth was the most extravagant gesture of all — a true act of contrition on his part for an incident which shook our marriage to the core.

Richard and I had put both boys down for Rugby when they completed their early schooling at Haileybury Junior in Windsor. I was unhappy with the concept of boarding in general, and worried about them being so far from home. I convinced Richard that Eton — just on our doorstep — would be less disturbing to the boys and to me. Richard agreed and said he would take the necessary steps to register the boys, although at this late stage there was only a slight chance they would be accepted unless they were accepted for a specific house by a specific master. I was more optimistic than he because the boys had an excellent school record and some of our friends who were masters at Eton were anxious to help.

Richard went off to renegotiate our agreement with the American franchisor and to discuss a possible joint project involving Weight Watchers food production in England.

While he was away I was accosted by a perplexed neighbour who was puzzled, and questioned me about the application which Richard had submitted on behalf of our sons to Eton. She had seen this as it had been referred to her husband who was a new house master there. She explained that our sons (with whom she had celebrated Jewish holidays at our home as a guest) were listed on their application as being members of the Church of England. I told her there must be some mistake and she replied that there was no mistake at all, showing me a copy of the form Richard had completed.

I was shattered, and more unhappy than I thought I could ever be. I couldn't understand why he would do such a thing.

Perhaps it stemmed from Richard's own insecurity, a legacy of his own unhappy boarding-school days. His mother having remarried a non-Jew, Richard's ethnic origin and early affiliations were minimized. He was nevertheless placed in the Jewish house of a very famous English boarding school. The Jewish boys found it hard to accept him because he knew nothing about Jewish customs or traditions, while the non-Jewish boys spurned his overtures and taunted him with stereotypical references to Jews. In later life, he became determined to be accepted as a true British gentleman and spent most of his life exaggeratedly playing that role.

For me, this was perhaps the greatest crisis in our relationship. It bespoke deceit, arrogance, and a total dismissal of what Richard well knew to be my deepest feelings and values. I phoned Richard in New York and warned him not to come home. He sought out my mother, his long-time ally. I felt that the real punishment for his action was having to tell her, the sole survivor of a family which had perished as proud Jews in the Holocaust, that the father of her grandchildren seemed ashamed of his heritage and had put her grandsons down for school as members of the Church of England.

My mother amazed me. She herself had never recovered from the slaughter of all who were closest to her and yet, for 'Shalom Beit' (harmony in the home), she agreed to come to England with Richard to help us through this crisis. Together, she and Richard arranged for me to consult a respected rabbi whom we all loved and revered, and who had been drawn to Richard in the past because of his wit and humour. The rabbi's counsel helped achieve a reconciliation but he warned me: 'Whatever hurts and confusions have gone into making Richard what he is, he is afraid of looking into himself, and certainly is not prepared to change. There will be more of these games played throughout your life together.'

He was right. Now Richard's 'games', his indirection, became more obvious to me and I began to notice this pattern even in the way he ran Weight Watchers. Things were never really the same again between us. Although there remained a powerful love which lasted even after our divorce, our differences in this and other areas where values were paramount kept adding scars and pouring acid on an open wound.

Richard believed that Gable House would be the solution to all our differences. It would certainly solve some problems for him. He had tried very hard indeed to run the business with Leslie but admitted partial defeat in the Weight Watchers food project. Moreover, he was now bored with the business and wanted something to do that had no connection with Weight Watchers. As a salve to his own wounds, Richard badly needed to indulge the Medici in him. Decorating a stately home would, in his eyes, clearly establish him as a country gentleman, a man of leisure and means, far removed from the more sordid world of business.

It would also be a fortress in which he could hide me away and separate me from all our acquaintances and friends. In the past they all used to drop in at our home in Datchet. At Gable House, he told my mother, he could 'lock Bernice away and just enjoy her'.

Gable House had been built by the Bowes-Lyons family and compared to our home in Datchet, which was comfortable but modest, it was luxurious to say the least. It had six bedrooms and three reception rooms, one of which was an elegant double drawing-room. Downstairs there was also a breakfast room for family meals, a kitchen, which we had modernized, a study, a music room and two cloakrooms. The children had their own playroom upstairs and Richard converted the attic so that he could store wine there. Outside was a patio and dining area, and there was a separate three-bedroomed house for the couple who acted as housekeeper and butler. We had a swimming pool and a tennis court, and best of all (and quite my favourite) there was a wonderful tree house for the children which Richard had designed himself.

We moved in early in 1972. Richard loved the house, and

hired David Hicks's firm to do the interior design. He wanted every last detail to be perfect and nothing was too much trouble. But I had as much as I could handle between three small children and the business, without trying to become the lady of the manor as well. I didn't want the extra responsibility the house represented. I didn't want to move and I never felt at home there.

Gable House was beautiful, but to me it seemed almost like a fortress. Our friends were so overwhelmed by our lavish entertaining there that they never invited us back because they felt they couldn't reciprocate on the same level.

Besides, Richard and I still had not solved the basic problem in our relationship: we still found each other exciting, we still loved each other, but we had never built up any communication on a deep and real level. There was still a satisfying, warm, physical attraction between us but there was a total vacuum as far as exchanging private thoughts and feelings. Our arguments increased in frequency and intensity, and our understanding and appreciation of one another and of our differences diminished.

On top of this, the pressures of work seemed to grow daily. Weight Watchers had kept me sane, it had brought me into contact with other women to whom I could relate, and with the professional and business people who cared about public health and wanted to improve it. Yet at the same time the organization was going through a difficult stage in its growth and as a result I was seeing less and less of the people who really mattered — the lecturers and the members. I was redirected into giving interviews, doing television shows and speaking in public. I was forced to read charts and yet more charts — discuss profitability, cash-flow and future expenditure. I felt I was moving further and further away from the very things that gave me joy and were most meaningful to me. It was exhausting and I made it even more so by coming home, no matter how far away it was, or how late the hour, in order to be with my children as much as possible.

Although I was unaware of it, Richard had already decided that the answer to all our problems was simple: sell Weight Watchers. He had even made the first moves towards this when I was pregnant with Alesia, although nothing came of his plans at the time.

I loved Weight Watchers. I needed it. It gave to me as much as I gave to it. It had filled an enormous gap in my life. I wasn't fully conscious of all this at the time — but I knew that I wasn't prepared to give it up. In any case, I felt, deep down, that if Richard and I were left with too much time on our hands, alone together, we would simply tear each other apart.

On the other hand — although I would never have agreed to the sale of Weight Watchers (at that stage because it would have really hurt me to see someone else running my 'baby') — I was not averse to the idea of our going public, so we began to explore the possibilities. I thought it might be a good move. Richard would be free to do whatever he wanted with his shares, even sell out and go back to the law or enter politics; and I could raise money to finance projects which would help me expand Weight Watchers further into health spas, diet holidays, magazines, books, cooking schools. When a famous health spa was up for sale, I hoped to buy it so that we could turn it back to its great days under its famous founder — and modernize it as well for Weight Watchers holidays, where executives would feel more comfortable than at our weekly classes.

However, there were problems. I dug my heels in and insisted on giving our staff and all our lecturers a shareholding in the proposed company; the financial advisers came up with legal and technical reasons why I couldn't do that but I insisted they find a way to have our dedicated staff share in a success they helped to create. In the event the economic climate changed, and Weight Watchers seemed suddenly less attractive to the stockbrokers. Nothing came of the idea.

By now Richard and I were in daily disagreement and I

began to fear that nothing could save our marriage. Our unhappiness had become so acute that we could not hide it; it was distressing us, confusing the children and hurting so many people who loved us. I remembered my own unhappiness as a child, listening to the heated disagreements about business between my parents, the two people I truly loved and admired, burying my head under the pillow each night so I could shut out the hurtful things they said to each other. I could not bear to subject our children to that. Anything was better than that — or so I thought.

I felt that it would be better to separate from Richard. At least the children could have peace when they were either with Richard or with me; they would no longer feel torn by their allegiances. I thought they would understand that we still loved each other, but that we could no longer live together. And I thought that if we separated, I could have some space, some life of my own and I would be able to introduce the children to the things I valued: museums, concerts, art.

At first I asked Richard if he would move out for several months so that I could sort myself out, but he refused. He had promised before we moved into Gable House that if things between us ever broke down, he would not force me to be the one to leave with the children. He even executed an agreement to that effect, drafted by his lawyer. But he went back on his word with no embarrassment. I took the children to Scotland for a holiday and then took them back to school while I went to Gable House, collected the things we needed and moved into a small hotel near Windsor. I thought I could live there without disturbing the children's schooling and still be close to our office, but it wasn't very convenient.

By this time much of my work seemed to centre on London. I was having meetings with Reader's Digest who were investigating the possibility of publishing a large 'coffee table' Weight Watchers cookery book. We were also preparing our first *TV Times* Weight Watcher of the Year promotion, and I was personally running a class for the *TV Times* staff so that they might write honestly as well as enthusiastically about their experiences.

Weight Watchers needed a London base and I needed a place from which to conduct my PR affairs — it would be less expensive than the rental of public rooms for cooking demonstration, press conferences, promotions and even training sessions. We were spending vast sums on hotels for overnight accommodation, meals and travel.

Up until this time I had only signed two cheques as a director of Weight Watchers (on both occasions when Richard was away and immediate payment was necessary). Gable House had consumed my savings, and I had neither a bank account nor cash. An old friend in whom I confided was outraged. He told me to write a Weight Watchers cheque as a deposit for the first two months rent for suitable quarters in London. I actually felt like a thief signing a company cheque but was encouraged to do so after consultation with my legal advisers.

The children and I moved into 12 Park Street, Mayfair, with my secretary, public relations assistant, and the cooks who were testing recipes for my third book. It was the best investment Weight Watchers had made in a long time.

Park Street saw the beginning of one successful Weight Watchers project after another, and even more successful promotions which helped keep Weight Watchers in the public eye. We soon became part of British folklore. Everyone forgot we were only six years old. It seemed as if we had always been there.

Our flat provided excellent kitchens for our cooks and the recipes could be tested and then brought immediately to the Good Housekeeping Institute where they were re-tested and confirmed on the spot. At Gable House I had only been allowed into the kitchen on my housekeeper's day off.

We could invite the press to lunch and show them how everything was done. We could hold training sessions and use in-house video, and lecturers and supervisors visiting from far away could stay overnight if necessary.

From the first, living in London was magical. I had almost forgotten that I was a born city girl and how hard it had been for me to leave exciting New York City with its vast array of cultural and entertainment opportunities. I enjoyed being at the centre of things again. I could take the children to Covent Garden, or to Billingsgate early in the morning to buy fruit and vegetables or fish. We bicycled everywhere and took walking tours around London, and visited the museums, art galleries and zoos, and attended children's concerts, and the ballet and special educational programmes. If it was announced that the BBC were going to broadcast a live concert from the Albert Hall, I didn't have to listen to the radio — the children and I could bike over and attend in person.

We launched the *TV Times* Weight Watcher of the Year from the flat and also celebrated the publication of my third book — the guest list was impressive and the event glamorous and successful. Richard insisted upon being present in some way: he sent a flower arrangement which was so large it dwarfed our vast drawing-room, looking more funereal than festive.

But generally everything seemed to be coming together and at last I had peace of mind, privacy, and a vast playground to share with my friends, fellow lecturers and supervisors at Weight Watchers, and with my children. Alesia attended a happy school and took ballet lessons while the boys came up from Windsor most weekends, and together we turned Hyde Park into a back garden. Life had become fun again!

CHAPTER EIGHT

For a while after I left Gable House in 1973, Richard and I met at board meetings and only at board meetings. The situation wasn't easy for the people who worked for Weight Watchers. At first, Richard kept his sphere of influence confined to financial and administrative matters, but then he began to involve himself in PR, promotion and training; he started to countermand my instructions and upset the balance we had carefully created with our division of labour.

He was still determined to sell Weight Watchers because he saw it as a rival for my affections. When I wouldn't agree to a sale, he felt the only solution was to destroy what we had built. He claimed and truly convinced himself it was a rival for my affections and believed we could not be a happy family with Weight Watchers. I decided to apply for a divorce.

On the day of the hearing, I had to enter the court via the basement in order to avoid the crowds of journalists; but there was no avoiding the press coverage. The sub-editors, of course, were unable to resist such headlines as: 'Founder of Weight Watchers Loses 19 Stone in One Day.'

But again, despite the divorce, Richard and I were still brought together through Weight Watchers. There were all kinds of projects to be discussed: magazines, new cook books, kitchen accessories designed by Terence Conran, the annual *TV Times* Weight Watcher of the Year Competition, and the development of new food products. Planning ahead on that scale was never my forte whereas Richard was marvellous at that kind of thing. We had worked so well together in the beginning because he was wonderful to bounce new ideas off and had helped me create memorable promotions. But after the divorce he was no longer interested. He resisted all my new ideas for taking Weight Watchers forward into health farms, magazines, expanding our health holidays, and most of all he was against the idea of extending our training methods by introducing New Age philosophy. As a result, there were board disagreements about the future direction of Weight Watchers.

After our divorce, I hoped to have more time to spend with the children, but that simply didn't happen. Increasingly, there seemed to be more drudgery and less fun in my life. The effect on the children worried me most — the boys' schooling suffered and they seemed withdrawn and unlike themselves.

It must have been confusing for them: it was confusing for us. Richard knew that without a Get, a Jewish divorce (which he would not grant me), I still felt married to him, and certainly my parents considered us legally married — and treated us thus — particularly when we were in the States.

Meanwhile, Richard never ceased to hope and plan for the sale of Weight Watchers and continued to hawk around the presentation which showed our financial position in the hope of finding a potential buyer. I was still trying to fight the sale, which could not go ahead without my consent, but my life soon became a round of meetings with lawyers, accountants and other business advisers who seemed uninterested in Weight Watchers other than as a product to be made more financially attractive to anyone who might be interested in buying it.

Even Leslie Levonton was won over by Richard and together they hired expensive outsiders whose job was to cut costs and improve efficiency, but who cared little for the heart of the business or for the people who made that heart beat. Richard began spending less and less time at the office and the administration fell more and more on me. Added to my own workload, it was just too much. Eventually I realized that Richard was never going to let the idea of selling Weight Watchers go; the business would be damaged and it would suffer.

It was then that I decided to initate negotiations with Weight Watchers International to buy us out. I felt that Jean Nidetch's dream remained pure; that Al Lippert, Weight Watchers' Chairman, lived Weight Watchers day and night and if he sold the company, it would be to someone wise enough to keep the original flame burning. (That someone proved to be the Heinz Corporation, who did, in fact keep the original management in place). At the same time, I knew that I could not bear to stay in Britain and watch someone else minding 'my baby'. Then negotiations faltered and I found myself all packed up with no place to go.

Richard came up with a proposal: he suggested I moved to Switzerland, a country where we had spent many happy holidays in the past, and which we both loved. I could put the children in schools near the house so that they could be home each night with me: I could be a full-time mother and in my spare time work on a new *Continental Diet Cookery Book.* He spoke with renewed enthusiasm about running Weight Watchers himself with the occasional visit from me to do some PR work and goodwill tours. He promised to lose weight and to be the breadwinner. The children were excited and secretly hoped that a new shared home would mean a reconciliation between their parents. I was exhausted and yearned for peace and, more than anything, I wanted the boys out of boarding school and in a family environment. Torn by all these feelings, I too allowed myself to hope that some kind of reconciliation would evolve.

We moved to Villars-sur-Ollon in April 1976 and after a spell in a hotel settled in Chalet Eglantine as a family with a daddy working in England and visiting at weekends. That was certainly how the community saw us. We Westons saw it as a new beginning. But Richard soon resumed negotions for the sale of the business, and finally completed the deal with Weight Watchers International. The Americans were the only people prepared to buy the company and run it without me. Every other potential buyer said that in

Britain, Weight Watchers and I were synonymous, and wanted me as part of the deal. Only the Americans had the experience and expertise to go it alone, and could incorporate British Weight Watchers into their worldwide organization. But there was more to it than that: the Americans were keen to buy us because, of all the franchisees, we were the only one with the right to produce our own food. They wanted to complete their own almost worldwide sale to Heinz, but Heinz wanted to buy the British market as well. In the end that was what happened and in 1978 the Heinz Company bought Weight Watchers worldwide.

In May I wrote a personal message to all my lecturers. I explained, 'For my own good and indeed for the sake of the future development of the business, I have to bow out of full-time involvement. As of this week, Weight Watchers International have become in a true sense the parent of the British Organization.'

As part of the original agreement with the Americans I agreed to do public appearances and to present awards. I carried on some activity for the Company for a short while, but it seemed wiser to us to eliminate any potential problem of divided or confused loyalties.

The contracts for the sale were sent to Geneva Airport for me to sign and return by courier. It was a totally impersonal ending, but the sadness and loss I felt as I signed my name was only the precursor of the sadness I was to feel and the losses I was to suffer in the very near future.

In June 1976 my father came to stay and I was able to spend quality time with him. Although in the past he had had two severe heart attacks, he had lost weight a long time ago and seemed fit and healthy. We had a particularly nice time together; he enjoyed the children and they responded to him. I felt for the first time that I was beginning to see the man behind the father, and I loved and respected this man. It was worth the pain of selling Weight Watchers to have this quiet, valued time with him. At the beginning of July we went to Geneva together, to see the children off to England because they were going to spend time with Richard. I then planned to write the *British Weight Watchers Story* and close that chapter with a tribute to the British women with whom I had been honoured to work.

Poppa and I went sightseeing. He was thrilled to see the places where Theodore Herzi had held the first Zionist congress, and the beautiful scenery of Geneva. We had a marvellous time. The hotel where we were staying did not have two single rooms, so we shared a suite. During the night I heard my father get up, and called out to him. He told me to go back to bed, but then I heard a strange sound, like a gasp or gurgle. When I went into his room he had collapsed and I couldn't rouse him. I rang for help and began to give him artificial respiration; it seemed to me that when I breathed in, he breathed back. The police arrived and told me he was dead, but I wouldn't believe it. I kept on breathing into his mouth. Then the ambulance men arrived and took over, but it was no use. They raced him to hospital, but my father was already gone.

To bring his body back to New York for an immediate burial and to lessen my mother's pain was all I could think of. It was a question of cutting through all the red tape in obtaining the necessary Swiss and American documents, since according to his religious beliefs he had to be buried the very next day. I called Richard because I knew if anyone could arrange it, he could. I will never forget how marvellous he was at this time. He handled all the tedious details and flew with me when I took my father's body home. He succoured me, comforted my mother and stood up proudly with us as a member of the family in the funeral home, receiving all our friends and relations during the mourning period with great courtesy and care.

My father's death left a gap in my life, but it was a comfort knowing that it had been swift, that he had had such a happy last day and had died without pain. Richard was supportive and caring and I couldn't have managed without him. We became lovers again.

Perhaps, as with so many women, my way of mourning was subconsciously to try to create life. As I look back, I understand how unfair this was to Richard. He could never understand that my sexual response to him wasn't in doubt, but it was only one facet of our relationship. Although we could be intimate and close, in many ways we still remained as far apart as ever in terms of what we wanted from life. Looking back I realize how much that must have hurt and confused him. At the time, it was not easy to be so objective.

After the sale of Weight Watchers, to distract myself from thoughts of my father's death and my own loneliness, I decided to stay in Switzerland and pick up the threads of my business career. Before I left London I had worked with Gus Arcon of Gym 'N' Tonic. Gus had invented the Platform Gym, a specialized piece of equipment which could turn any room into a gymnasium. It came as a complete package, measuring 22 ft by 6 ft, with mirrors, carpet and all the equipment you needed for a complete gym workout. There was a cycling machine, a ballet rail with a exerciser, a sit-up board and a pressure bar, as well as a Powerjog running machine. The easy to follow colour code, diagrams and instructions allowed people to follow their own personal 15- to 20-minute circuit. These machines were sold to the Holiday Inn chain of hotels in the UK and were a huge success. I decided to introduce them into hotels in Switzerland and later to other parts of Europe; they could be used not merely by overnight guests, but as part of a total health holiday package.

I then decided to form a new company called Slim-Fit. It incorporated all my experience in nutrition, dieting and behaviour modification together with my new interests in exercise, disease prevention, and the enhancement of health through special holidays.

I worked with Swiss gymnasiums and beauty clubs, teaching nutrition and the importance of a healthy diet to

people who were not fat, but also not fit; their prior
approach had been only to take physical exercise, but now
they wanted information on nutrition. I also brought overweight people to the gyms and health clubs for the very first
time; hitherto they had been afraid of looking ridiculous in
front of the 'jocks' who made them feel self-conscious.

For these people I devised a programme of simple gym exercise with and without equipment under very careful supervision.

I became very interested in aquathinics and hydro-
aquatics — exercises that could be done in water. I found
that the sheer buoyancy of the medium made fat people feel
lighter, happier, and less worried about their weight. Water
induced a feeling of relaxation and enjoyment which made
it easier to overcome the normal fears fat people have about
what they look like while exercising.

I worked with people who were on holiday and had time
to think about improving their health; and I worked with
businessmen, encouraging them to lose weight and think
healthy while they were taking part in conferences or
management training courses.

I became increasingly interested in the importance of
exercise and the ways in which overweight people could
incorporate it into their lives. I felt it unfortunate that our
Weight Watchers classes were held in places where there
was no space to include exercise of any kind.

In the very early days of Weight Watchers we knew little
about the value of exercise. We accepted what some American nutritionists taught, namely that you had to walk 79
miles to lose a pound (the implication being that it wasn't
worth the effort). But over the years we learned that taking
regular exercise improves your metabolic rate and the
efficiency with which your body burns fat. Weight Watchers
did recommend exercise, then, but could not deal with it
within its operations.

I discovered in Switzerland that when you take only
limited exercise you are more limited in what you may eat,
and the amount you may eat — the body working less

efficiently in burning calories. In addition, a purely nutritional approach to weight loss overlooks the pyschological satisfaction to be derived from exercising: you are less likely to head for the biscuit tin out of boredom!

On the other hand it was not my intention to make joggers out of obese people who hardly moved or walked anywhere. I was not nor am I now an advocate of vigorous aerobic activity for inexperienced people. I have seen too many injuries as a result of such exercises. In my experience at Weight Watchers classes, members came to class carrying anything from 20 pounds to 20 stone of extra weight. It was a natural reaction to want to put that package down often, so eventually they virtually stopped moving altogether.

At Slim-Fit we took these immobile fatties and let them 'play' in the gyms; but I watched carefully because I knew gym teachers might push them too fast or too hard.

Founding Slim-Fit involved me in much research. Apart from finding out as much as I could about aerobic exercise, anaerobic exercises, jogging, etc, I had to familiarize myself with European eating habits which were quite different from British ones. Europeans use meal-times as social occasions. Also, attitudes towards weight vary from country to country. Whereas it is important (in terms of social status) for a French woman to be slim, that is not necessarily so for Italian women. Europeans tend to be less interested in the hows and whys of human behaviour; the psychology of eating is less interesting to them than it might be to Americans or the British.

In effect, I was introducing a totally new concept once again by talking about behaviour modification. Moreover, Europeans had yet to accept the fact that obesity was a killing disease. They lagged behind for many years in that respect.

Even the way in which Swiss classes were organized was different. In Britain there was something homely about Weight Watchers. A lecturer could stick up a handwritten card in a doctor's surgery or a newsagent's window giving details of the local class and people would come. But in

Switzerland everything had to be expensively produced or packaged otherwise people just were not interested. People were far more likely to invest a substantial sum in a course of classes than to turn up and pay a weekly fee.

I also became very interested in alternative health therapies such as Touch for Health, and brought practitioners from Belgium and England to the Eurotel in Villars. In these courses we taught that there is a flow of energy through your body which, if trapped, causes a great deal of stiffness, pain and illness. By teaching people to change their mental attitude, and by using a form of acupressure, we taught them to release the flow and improve their health. Back pain and tight shoulders were our speciality treatment. Margaret Brazier Estevez, our nanny, qualified at the Champney's Beauty School and returned to add massage, aromatherapy and other beauty and alternative health therapies.

Inner ski-ing holidays were another success. I was introduced to Tim Gallway who had developed a theory that in any sport there was both an outer game and an inner game; it was the inner game which always defeated you. The only way to 'win' was to free yourself from your inner fears.

He wrote a book called *The Inner Game*, which was later adapted to cover tennis, golf and ski-ing. Together with some friends and business acquaintances, I helped organize the first Inner Ski-ing Holiday in Kitzbühl, Austria, where we all learned to overcome our fears and relax — and did learn to ski better.

Another project was a tie-in with the management courses run by the Harvard Business School at the Mirador Club in Montpelier, above Vevey. The Mirador was a superb country club, but also the headquarters of Harvard in Europe to which executives from different countries would come for eight-week intensive management courses. The courses were testing and stressful, and the participants worked flat out; throughout the men who attended them ate and drank heavily, the way men do when they are on expense accounts. I had heard that several men had suffered heart attacks after attending these courses — and I wasn't surprised. They took no exercise, ate unwisely, and were under constant stress.

I used to take my children to the Mirador to swim, and during our visits I often talked to the executives who were also using the pool. On one occasion I began a conversation with the chairman of a large UK bank who was close to retirement. He confessed that he was frightened; he believed that once he retired, he would simply die. He told me that over the years, as he had become more and more successful in his career, he had grown apart from his wife. She felt unable to keep up with him or to act as his hostess. As a result he had begun to do more and more of his entertaining away from home and had spent less and less time with her. He had no hobbies and felt that retirement offered him nothing to look forward to for the future. He told me he would have liked to start communicating with his wife again but didn't know how.

It was obvious that a great many businessmen faced the same kind of problems. I started to think about developing programmes for executives which would combine exercise, healthy eating, stress reduction, personal communication skills and advice on how to develop new areas of interest: all of this tied in with what we had created in British Weight Watchers. It had become something much more than just a weight loss organization which aided people to shed pounds; I had become particularly interested in what women as well as men did *after* they lost weight, the way they directed the new energy they had developed.

Just as we had helped formerly fat people in Weight Watchers to blossom by encouraging them to experiment with clothes and make-up, just as we had given them new skills in managing their lives, just as we had given them a new confidence to go off in new directions, so I began to see that Slim-Fit could offer these and other new opportunities to men as well as women — and to people who were not necessarily fat.

We soon began self-improvement courses, and our health programme ran alongside the management courses; we held individual counselling sessions as well as group discussion in the evenings. Instead of swapping stories about cars or work or women, the men would talk about retirement, bereavement, fears of death or old age and other issues which dearly concerned them. The courses were very successful: many of the men lost weight as well, eating my diet menus developed especially for the hotel or for the conference, and they felt better than they had for years.

Slim-Fit was beginning to grow and I could take pride in it. I also hoped that it would secure my financial future and enable me to support my children as well. Richard's parallel investments were turning out to be costly, and in one serious instance disastrous. He now felt he was unable to contribute financially to the children's schooling.

The lease on the first house in Switzerland having terminated, we moved to another. This was called Shangri-La — a place of no care. If only it could have been so! The location was certainly magical. From every window there were spectacular views of the Dents du Midi mountains, and the children and I woke up every morning to the sound of cow bells.

Yet that period of my life seemed shrouded in confusion: I was muddled about my feelings for Richard, torn between my need to be a mother and my need to work.

As if the traumatic loss of my father hadn't been enough of a blow, I was called to America again and learned that my mother was seriously ill with cancer; her treatment consisted of a series of chemotherapy treatments and I began to fly regularly back and forth to America to be with her. For the first time she needed me and I wouldn't fail her. My reason for agreeing to the sale of Weight Watchers was to have my children at home with me: now I realized I had paid that price for nothing. Because I was away so much, it became necessary for the boys to be boarders after all.

In January 1977 we were together again as a family in

America. Because of my mother's illness, we decided to hold Douglas's bar mitzvah in Miami. As far as my mother was concerned, Richard and I were still husband and wife. She didn't recognize the civil divorce and didn't bother (or want) to tell our American family about it. Douglas's great day was a joyous occasion, spiritual and moving — and we all tried to make things as happy as possible for my mother. Douglas was brilliant, and Richard and I were proud and so happy.

Unfortunately, after Douglas returned to Switzerland he became ill and eventually a psychologist told us that he was under great stress — trying to re-unite his parents. Once again, I was forced to face the fact that the problems which existed between Richard and me were causing problems for the children. I was stricken with guilt and willing to try anything to sort things out once and for all. We began family therapy, but it proved too great a strain for Douglas, disturbed Graeme and confused Alesia. Richard and I were advised to start a courtship which we had never had, and to get to know one another. We had the time: no business, no distractions. After a short 'honeymoon,' however, a distraction did appear.

By the end of the year Richard had become a fully licensed pilot, bought his own airplane and taken a flat just over the French border in Divonne. He hoped to build a new career for himself in aviation.

In 1976, two planes, a British Airways Trident en route from London to Istanbul and an Inex-Adria DC9 flying from Split to Cologne, had collided in mid-air over Zagreb, Yugoslavia. Everyone on board both planes was killed: the 54 passengers and crew on the Trident and the 108 passengers and five crew on the DC9. Richard had earlier been dating one of the hostesses on that Trident, and since they had become quite close, he represented her family at the subsequent trial of the Yugoslavia air traffic controllers which took place in May 1977.

During the trial it became clear that one man, Gradimir Tasic, was being made the scapegoat for the inadequacies of

the system. It emerged that they were four men under-
strength, the equipment was inadequate, and training facilities were bad. Infuriated by the injustice, Richard changed
sides during the trial and through a Yugoslav lawyer made
an impassioned plea for the defence. Despite this, Tasic was
given a seven-year sentence for 'causing' the crash, but
Richard refused to give up and embarked on a one-man
campaign to secure his release.

I was in the court in Zagreb to provide moral support
and was thrilled with Richard's stand. The judge invited us
into Chambers and spoke to us as colleagues. I used my PR
talents and phoned the local *Times* correspondent in
Belgrade. She wrote a marvellous report about Richard
which was picked up by wire services all over the world. He
became a media star and a hero to many people in the
aviation world.

Richard wrote me the most beautiful love letter,
promising a whole new future. We attended a celebration
party together in London at the home of a British Air Vice-
Marshal. I was thrilled to see Richard honoured by so
many and his plans to improve air traffic control procedures
applauded. Richard whispered: 'See, I'm watching what
I'm eating — I want to be on my best form.' It was heaven.

Then, on leaving, our hostess asked if I would sign her
visitors' book. I was a celebrity, she said — she had been a
Weight Watcher and I had given her an award in the past.
Richard's face clouded over. He was quiet and subdued as
we left. Then, as if a clap of thunder exploded, he shouted:
'That's it — she never asked me to sign her visitors' book,
and I've been there five times. Weight Watchers will always
be there — it will always spoil things for me!' He raced off
and left me standing in the street, alone and confused. No
exploded balloon ever came down so fast or felt so flat.

For the first time in a long while, I needed Richard more
than he needed me. I wanted to be with him, support his
cause, share this valuable new career which, for the first
time, gave his life special meaning. But here I was,

excluded. There was more pain to come.

In June 1978, my mother died. Her death hit me far harder than my father's had done. I had been through so much with her during her illness. She had been so brave, endured so much. She seemed to have pulled through after a major, painful operation. Her death happened so quickly that I could not say goodbye to her. An experimental drug took away her speech, weakened her, and may well have hastened her death. At least she died in the loving warmth of my sister's home.

I mourned her, not just for myself but for Richard as well. The love he felt for her and the unqualified love she gave him was the most meaningful relationship he ever had. Through all our ups and downs it had always been my mother who had brought us back together. She was the bridge between us, and now she was gone. After her funeral, Richard and I knew this was a turning point for us.

Now we began to try to make new lives for ourselves. Through me Richard had met an American woman and her daughter, Polly, who lived just down the valley. Polly went to work for Richard and later became his girlfriend. I was pleased: I felt Richard needed someone in his life, and, to be honest, I hoped that now he would be less likely to interfere in mine.

I became very close to a psychiatrist called Klaus Hertzeneed. Since my divorce I had dated very few men, and all those relationships had been platonic. With Klaus it was different. I enjoyed being with him. He was funny, intellectual, understanding, and oh so very gentle and kind.

We talked about making a future together — marrying and setting up a temporary part-time residence in Jerusalem. He would still continue with his Swiss practice and I would run Slim-Fit until I could sell it and recoup my heavy investment. Klaus cautioned me not to discuss these plans with the children or anyone. He was concerned that there would be trouble from Richard.

Needing extra finance for Slim-Fit, I struck a deal with

an English investor and introduced him to my associates, particularly a couple who were friends of Richard's and mine. Everything seemed to be going well and I was relieved and happy.

I had planned to spend Christmas in South Africa with Klaus, meeting his family. I asked Richard to take the children on holiday. He agreed, but on the eve of my departure he called and delayed our arrangements. I couldn't leave and Klaus was crestfallen. He had made so many plans.

Tragically, on New Year's Eve he was involved in a car crash which left him paralysed. I heard nothing about it at first and thought he was angry with me for putting the children before him. His mother then called and explained and we all agreed to fly to Israel together where we hoped for some treatment, some miracle cure.

While I was there, Richard decided to wreck Slim-Fit. He encouraged the English businessman and the friendly couple to join forces. Together with Richard, they informed all my employees that I was not coming back and that they were the new owners of Slim-Fit.

They moved all my files and equipment out of our office and set up in competition with me. I was forced to initiate legal action against them; Richard prepared their case, resulting in a trial which effectively destroyed what had been a budding business with great potential. Another victory for Richard — but why?

I could never understand why he wanted to do this; at first I did not believe it possible that he had. Only now, perhaps in retrospect, can I see that my being in any way in control of a diet business again 'threatened him' in some way, and made him feel he would never be able to rid himself of the Weight Watchers stigma. He feared even his new career in aviation would not wipe out his reputation as the 'Weight Watchers man'.

Whatever his motives, there now seemed little to keep me in Switzerland.

Douglas seemed unhappy in the Swiss school. Richard

and I had agreed to send him to a summer school in America to see if he would prefer schooling in the States. Klaus was also going to America for special treatment.

In July I flew to Boston, to visit Douglas at school, planning to stop first to see Klaus in hospital. The flight was delayed and I arrived physically shattered. I rented a hire car at the airport — a sports car of some kind. On the dark and unfamiliar road, I hit a curb. The car leapt into the air, rolled over and over, finally coming to rest upside down on the driver's side. I was lucky not to have been killed.

As it was, I ended up with stitches in my head, fragments of glass in my eye and whiplash injuries to my neck and back. Heavily sedated, I was taken to my hotel near Douglas's school. I phoned Klaus. He sounded quiet — but I could sense he was upset and disappointed. It was the last time we spoke.

To this day I'm not certain what really happened. I know that the medical prognosis for his recovery had dashed his hopes of ever regaining movement in his legs. There was unlikely to be any further improvement. I knew he was looking forward to seeing me. Yet the next day his mother rang me to break the news that he had committed suicide.

Why did he do it? All I remembered was how brave and patient he had been — how optimistic. Yet he was also a realist and he made his own choices.

The thought of making a new home in Israel became more and more attractive. I had been through a love affair with a man who wanted it as our home and now I suddenly felt a need for Israel — a nurturing environment like my Brooklyn past and a welcoming future where I could escape finally from whatever hold Richard still had over my emotions. It was also the one place he would not be anxious to follow me.

Richard now took unilateral action and placed Douglas in Gordonstoun School in Scotland. Since we had joint custody of the children I could have challenged his actions but this would have meant a legal battle and I simply couldn't subject Douglas to that. It seemed better to accept that Douglas and Graeme should have the education Richard wanted for them while I would concentrate on trying to impart some of my own values to Alesia. I knew she loved Israel and would be happy to live with me there. But in order to do this I had to petition the British courts for a change in the original divorce agreement. Richard opposed my petition and thus began a battle which almost became my Waterloo.

Before the matter came to court, I decided once again to press Richard for a Jewish divorce. Under Jewish law only a man can divorce his wife: a wife has no rights in the matter. (I consider this to be one of the greatest injustices of my faith, and how intelligent women can accept this and remain loyal to orthodox practices, I cannot understand, but it would take another book to do justice to my feelings on this subject.) Under Israeli law, our British divorce was null and void, so obtaining Richard's co-operation in this was vital to my plans.

Richard and I met in London to discuss the matter and although he had always refused my requests for a Get (the Rabbinical Court divorce) in the past this time he agreed. I felt as if a huge weight had been lifted from me and suddenly everything seemed hopeful.

We went off to see our respective lawyers. Both sets of barristers and solicitors were due to meet to discuss various points in order to try to reach a settlement, rather than do battle in court. Richard seemed poised to allow me to take Alesia to Israel. In fact, by this stage, the Jewish divorce was the last hurdle left. As soon as I walked into my barrister's chambers, however, I could sense a change of atmosphere. It emerged that my lawyers had been given to understand that a real breakthrough had taken place but before the two sides met, Richard asked to see me personally.

I was puzzled, but agreed. At our meeting Richard began to talk about the future as if the entire slate had been wiped clean and as if my plans for Israel were nothing more than a whim. He suggested that we should remarry and go to America as a united family — settle in California where he had applied to take the bar exam, and would practise aviation law. We could put our children into day schools there and start a new life together. He invoked the memory of my mother and reminded me how pleased she would have been to see this happen.

I refused. I tried to explain that although I loved him, and though we had always been able to have spells of intense happiness together, our values were still different and I could not be his wife. We talked for a long time but I couldn't make him understand. Perhaps no one could. I finally realised that it would never be possible to reach an agreement with Richard that was meaningful; perhaps our troubles were as much my fault as his, but all I wanted to do was cut and run — and Israel was where Alesia and I wanted to be.

Richard left but his solicitor reappeared, while I was still sitting there, and announced to my counsel that they were 'going to come out fighting' — and fight they did.

Richard also changed his mind about the Jewish divorce and before the case came to court, rang me to say he was going to marry Polly in a civil ceremony. As a married couple they stood a better chance of getting custody of Alesia than I, as a single parent. If I wanted to go to Israel, I could, but not with her; and in Israel I was still his wife — the civil courts there had no jurisdiction over marital and custody matters.

In other circumstances I would have been pleased for Richard about his marriage but now it was just another tactic to browbeat me with.

The run-up to the hearing was indescribably harrowing as delay followed delay. Alesia was under pressure and Douglas and Graeme were forced to take sides. Graeme suddenly grew up and became a stalwart protector of his sister. I was fascinated and proud and very grateful.

Every time I flew into London to see my lawyers I was hit

by another surprise, another bombshell. I was permanently exhausted and worried. I felt vulnerable and alone, I couldn't sleep. A friend suggested I see her doctor who prescribed tranquilizers and sleeping pills. I couldn't eat and my weight dropped to below 100 pounds (7st 2lb). Gillian Rimmer, my PA of many years, told me she knew I was in trouble: 'If you can turn down scones and cream during afternoon tea at the Inn on the Park, then you aren't the lady I know!'

I felt as if I were on trial, and, in a way, I was. But it was more than that. It may be difficult to understand, but for Richard and me our civil divorce had never been as final as it is for most people; it was just a step along the way, merely confirming that I had the right to live separately. This hearing represented the real break and it was now that all the pain, the hurt — mud-slinging, if you will — took place. Any illusions I had about him were gone. If the divorce had opened a door for me, then this battle over Alesia gave me the chance to walk through and close it behind me.

The hearing lasted a week. Somehow I got through it, with the aid of friends, Gillian Rimmer, Virginia Levin and my Israeli cousin, Rikki. It was hard for me to feel optimistic about the outcome. The judge put me through a very tough cross-examination and didn't seem to comprehend why Richard's counter-proposal for Alesia to attend Benenden School in England did not please me. All the worst aspects of my character were paraded. Worse still, the judge deferred his summing up and judgement until after the weekend. I was in such a state that I remember nothing about the following two days except that by the Monday morning I was convinced I would lose and have to appeal.

When it came to the summing up, the more I heard, the more convinced I was that I had lost. I was so emotionally drained that I forgot the one basic maxim that all lawyers learn: if the decision is going to go to X, the judge usually tries to make Y feel better by emphasising all his good qualities and by making the point that although X is far from perfect, what matters in the end is not who is good or who is bad, but what are the best interests of the child.

The more I heard, the more despairing I felt. The court swam before my eyes and I would have fainted if my solicitor's secretary had not grabbed me and whispered: 'Hold on. This is the best thing that could have happened because it means he is going to give you the decision.' And so he did.

But at that precise moment I felt far from victorious. I felt like a prize-fighter who had been knocked down just as the bell sounded — and then declared the winner on points. I was so punch drunk I could hardly take it all in.

Alesia and I arrived in Israel in the summer of 1980. It was a joyous time — all the friends we had made on our previous visit were in celebratory mood. Ulpan Akivah, the Hebrew Language School we both attended, was on the sea; there was singing and folk dancing in the evening, and relaxed classes with an extraordinary mix of young and old students from all over the world mingling together. There were Arabs, Jews, Druse sheikhs, Israeli nationals, Europeans and Americans.

Alesia and I were students together but she soon outstripped me in Hebrew; she was a natural linguist and even picked up bits of Arabic and enjoyed conversations with the Druse sheikhs. It was a heavenly time, but our newfound peace was of short duration.

Richard fulfilled the threats he had made at the trial of keeping me so busy with lawsuits that I couldn't rest easy in Israel. He caused the Swiss authorities to revoke the residence permits granted to the children and myself and froze all my bank accounts. I lived on my wits and little else for our first year — but it meant running back and forth to Switzerland and the UK almost constantly.

Still nothing could dim my joy. The boys arrived and with Alesia we toured Israel from north to south, going into the Sinai for safaris, sleeping on beaches along the Sea of Galilee and the Red Sea — protected always by our trusty

3½ pound Yorkshire Terrier, 'Duke'. The boys learned to
scuba dive and were adopted by the strangest assortment of
people. There were wide-eyed settlers of the West Bank,
young religious converts seeking to induct them into
Orthodox Jewry, irreverent but joyous rangers who took
them into the wilds and swimming with dolphins. There
was a retired general who filled them with stories of his
great tank battle campaigns of 1948, '56 and '67 — and
there were always musicians, poets, artists, statesmen,
anxious to share their joy and love of Israel. We were new
settlers, and the older settlers were determined that we
should stay. Each of them was determined to teach us what
Israel meant, but from their point of view.

After the trial, I was particularly thin; I was still having
difficulty weaning myself away from the extensive dosages
of tranquilizers and medication which saw me through the
court hearing and reduced the eye trouble I had developed
after my car crash. Despite everything, I was attractive and
'new' and soon found myself besieged and courted by
extremely desirable men. I felt very vulnerable alone with
Alesia and so I kept myself too busy to catch. Without Get,
the Jewish divorce which Richard still refused to grant, I
still felt married, as indeed I was according to Israeli law. As
a woman alone I was vunerable — happy, but a little uneasy.

I couldn't rest until Alesia entered school. Would she
really settle happily? Would the freedom and relaxed
atmosphere of Israeli schools confuse her after her formal
French-Swiss experience? Could Richard have been right?

On her first afternoon home from school she danced in,
the happiest I had ever seen her. 'Oh, Mummy, I've got
friends — the teachers are lovely, the headmaster lets us call
him by his first name, and I can study ballet in a real
Academy. Everything's so lovely, but *you* will have to serve
guard duty at the school like all the other parents.'

I had made the right decision after all, and it was all
worth it.

Living in Jerusalem is a gift in any case. It is one of the
most beautiful and sensual cities in the world. Looking out

across the Old City one sees the four major religious quarters, and smaller areas representing every other religion in the world; beyond that lies the desert, the valleys leading down to the Dead Sea with the mountains of Moab announcing the presence of Jordan. So much tragedy has been enacted in these streets, in these valleys and deserts, so many wars have been fought and so many lives lost, that one's own problems appear minute in contrast. The view from our balcony was a constantly changing picture; the City of Gold, as Jerusalem is called because of its extra-ordinary light, is the best 'upper' in the world.

Jerusalem is also a city where one meets everyone if you stay long enough. It is intellectually and artistically stimu-lating; there can be fifty concerts, art exhibitions and poetry readings going on, on any one night alone. One is never bored. It is a classless society. You could walk out of the lift of the hotel in which we lived to find your dog being petted by President Mitterand of France, or George Schultz in conversation about football with one of your favourite Arab waiters.

Very unusual friendships develop there. Alesia and I formed our earliest and warmest friendship with a young Palestinian who worked at the hotel; soon he was inviting us home for lunch to meet his family or to pick grapes from their orchards. We attended Greek Orthodox Easter services, had deep discussions with Franciscan monks, had our faces and clothes painted by one of the world's leading artists. Alesia used to say that she loved Jerusalem because each time her mother went out for a loaf of bread, she came back with someone exotic — such as a monk who had finished a vow of silence after twenty years and couldn't stop talking. In fact, everyone talked and when they talked they talked politics; everyone had a different point of view but was certain that God was on his side.

In 1982 war broke out in the Lebanon. Richard, responding to all the adverse, anti-Israeli agitation, decided that he no longer wanted Alesia to live in Israel. That summer, when she went to visit him in England, he used a family disagreement as an excuse not to allow her to return to Israel with me and placed her in a Church of England boarding school. He went back to court, obtained a temporary order setting aside the 1980 custody judgement, and prevented me from seeing her or communicating with her. I was swept away on a tide of anger, confusion and resentment. Like me, Alesia had bloomed in the friendly, free, accepting warmth of Israel; now she was confined to a highly disciplined boarding school. When I did manage to make contact with her through my friend and secretary Gillian Rimmer, Alesia told me she wanted to continue to live in Israel. I knew I had to find some way to have that decision overturned.

The first court action had been a nightmare but this one was many times worse. Newspapers and television were stridently anti-Israel; each time I turned on the radio or the television, the broadcasters and commentators were attacking the very essence of Israel's position in the world as a democratic nation. On the first day I appeared in court, as an American lawyer appearing without counsel and ex parte, I made reference to an Israeli judgement. Before I could continue the judge retorted, 'We in England don't think much of Israeli judgement at this moment.' The battle no longer seemed only to be over what was best for my child.

In the end I didn't win the case — Alesia did. She was prepared to stand up aged 11 and tell the court-appointed welfare officer that Israel was her home and she wanted to live there. The welfare officer who visited her was straight-thinking and unbiased. She reported back to the court that Alesia's best interests would be furthered by returning her to Israel.

Alesia could not return with me straight away but had to complete her English school term. Back in Israel I should have been happy but felt as if I were in a trance — lonely, experiencing great pain, having difficulty with my eyes. Without realizing it, I was literally 'hooked' on the tranquil-izers I had been taking to get me through the stressful court actions. I spent long days unable or unwilling to leave the house or even to answer the telephone. Most of my friends in Israel and abroad thought I was 'busy as usual' but in fact I was battling to wean myself off the medication and experiencing deep depression, anxiety and loneliness.

When I sought help, whether in England or in Israel, the doctors merely suggested a change in the strength of medication or the substitution of other pills. I soon learned that there were many women in the same situation. The old family doctors that I had known in my youth in Brooklyn had time for their patients. Modern doctors have neither their concerned approach nor that time. Perhaps it is easier for them to prescribe under the NHS or other health schemes, pills and palliatives to calm down 'nervy' women. When I first came to England, no matter what ailment a female patient complained of, she was usually advised to 'put her feet up', and have a cup of tea. Strangely enough, I think that was better advice than modern day prescriptions for Librium and Valium and the barbiturates, tranquilizers and mood-changing substances.

Again I resorted to group therapy and sought help from those who had experienced the same problems. They tried to help me wean myself off these medications and at least got me out of the flat. Jossi Stern, my constant companion and confidant, who had suffered much in his lifetime, was a comforting, loving and amusing friend, who helped by reminding me that Alesia was coming home soon and that was enough reason to pull myself together.

The following summer Richard flew to America to act as an expert witness at the hearing of another aviation disaster. Alesia went along with him on holiday. Richard always travelled first class, and according to Alesia, he tucked in to the airline meals with his usual gusto. When they arrived in Washington they had dinner at the hotel. The following morning he took her for his favourite American breakfast and then they went back to the hotel to rest again. Alesia fell asleep and awoke to hear her father talking on the phone; he was asking the hotel for a doctor. As he began to dial again, she saw him slump forward. Despite her efforts and those of the hotel staff, who gave him artificial respiration, they were unable to revive him. Alesia was taken off by ambulance with him; a nun was called in to administer the last rites — something that is done as a matter of course in America — and she comforted Alesia. Only then did she realize that her father was dead.

I had lost my father in almost identical circumstances, but I was a grown woman. Alesia was alone in a strange city, unable to reach any of the family. She adored her father. He had been a doting parent — indulgent and uncritical — and a playmate extraordinaire. Her courage was exemplary, her dignity beyond understanding in one so young. A kindly nurse was able to reach Alesia's tutor in Israel. She contacted Richard's brother, who informed the boys.

I was travelling to visit Bruna Latchman, a former Weight Watchers lecturer and friend, in England. On my arrival she asked me to ring Gillian, my personal assistant. As I began to dial she touched me gently and said, 'Bernice, I don't want you to hear this over the phone — Richard is dead.' I was in a trance. It was unbelievable. Suddenly I realized what she was saying about Alesia all alone in Washington and knew I had no time for my own feelings.

How can a mother describe what she feels about a 12-year-old child witnessing the death of a beloved father? There would be time later to come to terms with what this meant to me and the boys — my sons who patterned their every stance, intonation, manner upon their dynamic father. Where were they? How were they?

I pulled myself together and arranged for my niece and nephew to fly to Alesia at once, and began trying to arrange my own journey to Washington. After speaking to Graeme, I learned that Douglas was on his way to the airport. I raced to Heathrow to meet him but missed the plane. I was then able to speak to Alesia, who was now with her cousins and was being taken to my sister's house. She and Douglas indicated that they wanted to have their father's body brought home quickly to England for burial. Graeme concurred. I knew Richard's mother would want him home as well.

Richard's wife, Polly, was in Scandinavia and unreachable at that moment. I had to act quickly as I remembered Richard advising me to do when my father died. I telephoned the pathologist and convinced him to bypass all the red tape and help with the necessary certificates; I arranged to have Richard's body flown back on the same flight as Alesia and Douglas. I asked a rabbi who had been a friend of Richard's and mine to help with the funeral arrangements. He also agreed to officiate at the funeral.

I was later told that there was to be a cremation instead of a burial and was asked by Polly not to attend the ceremony. I respected her wishes and after a while returned with Alesia to Israel. Having put my feelings 'on hold', I suppressed them for a very long time.

With hindsight I can see only too clearly that the very differences which drew Richard and me together in the first place eventually drove us apart. My 'Americanism' made it easy for me to venture new approaches in business over here. The British were unable to pigeonhole me into a particular class or category and instead described me as 'exotic', 'unusual', 'original' or 'dynamic'. It was these very qualities that made Richard fall in love with me, just as it was his essential 'Englishness' which drew me to him. Although he was always creative, original and energetic, he packaged those talents into almost a caricature of a gentlemanly, eccentric Englishman.

What began as a game between us developed into almost a tug of war as to how we should live our lives and bring up the children. Once we were successful enough with Weight Watchers to be able to do more than simply keep our heads above water, once we could stop worrying about how to pay the mortgage and put the children through school, once we had time to spare to think about what else we wanted from life, the differences between us magnified.

Looking back, I can see I was almost totally without

sympathy for Richard's position. When he did things which ran counter to my beliefs I remembered past hurts and dishonesty and simply exploded with anger. Yet underneath, I was often hurt and frightened. I had been claustrophobic as a child and had learned to ameliorate it, but with a husband, children, a demanding business and no time for myself, I felt I couldn't breathe and had no one to talk to and share my fears with. So anger became a frequent release.

At the same time, I don't think I ever really appreciated how much Richard felt he had sacrificed in order to make Weight Watchers a success. He had been forced to choose between the business and being a partner in a prestigious law firm — and in choosing Weight Watchers he felt he had relinquished an essential part of his hopes and ambitions: the respect of his clients and peers, and his place as a part of the Establishment that he held so dear. I regret that at the time I had neither the sensitivity nor the real knowledge of his background to understand how deeply he was hurt or how bitterly he hated having to make such a choice.

Perhaps my expectations of marriage and of Richard were simply too high. All I know is that my yearning for intimacy — for caring and sharing — on a more than purely physical level was undernourished in our relationship and not surprisingly found an outlet only through Weight Watchers and not through our marriage. Through the business I was able to fulfil my family traditions of service to society — improving the world somewhat while sharing the highs, the lows, and the aspirations of our members. It was my own personal tragedy that I was successful with so many yet ultimately failed with Richard.

In a chance meeting in Israel a year later, the rabbi who officiated at Richard's funeral told me how sad he always felt when visiting the Golder's Green crematorium to see Richard's ashes in a dusty plastic bag on the floor — unclaimed and seemingly unwanted. I explained to the rabbi that I had no authority over Richard's remains and that my entreaties to those who did, to honour him in some way, went unheeded. I began having nightmares. The thought of ebullient, bombastic, life-loving Richard contained in a plastic bag on the floor seemed unbearable. It became almost an obsession that I should 'free him' from this ignominy.

I had promised the children and myself that I would remember only the 'good times'. The memories came flooding back. I remembered many good times; many joyous and wonderful times. I remembered especially how I had come to love him, how he had given me the attention I seemed to need which helped me grow from a fat girl from Brooklyn into the sophisticated 'woman of the world' he wanted me to be.

One day, when I felt despondent and tearful about all this, an English friend made a suggestion. 'Your Hungarian friend Jossi taught me a Hungarian saying: "A true friend is one with whom you would steal a horse." I will help you steal Richard's ashes.' He suggested that we write to Richard's widow and family advising them that I would inter his ashes in Israel with an appropriate memorial if they did not act to claim them.

By Israeli law, I was still Richard's widow and from that standpoint not without my rights. After a suitable period of time and discussion with Alesia, I selected a marvellous place in the Jerusalem Forest and dedicated a small park in his name near the Kennedy Memorial and the Arthur Rubenstein grave and monument; it was also not far from a playground where one could hear, in the distance, the happy voices of children at play.

I did hijack Richard's ashes and finally brought them to Jerusalem after a protracted and difficult journey. We finally put him to rest, not in a graveyard but in a 'happy' place, both dignified and beautiful. Alesia, her best friend, Jossi and I were there. After that I, too, began to feel at rest. I still have not yet been able to close the door on that relationship, but somehow, an enormous weight was lifted from my shoulders and heart.

CHAPTER NINE

One of the things that struck me about living in Israel in the eighties was how unhealthy the diet of many of its citizens had become. My first introduction to the country had been as a teenager in the late fifties when I lived for a while in Kibbutz Afikim in the Galilee. Meals there were frugal and sensible, consisting mostly of fresh fruit and vegetables produced by the kibbutz itself. Eating was not a ritual, dining was not a social occasion. You simply ate together in a communal hall, cleaned up cheerfully afterwards, and then walked or cycled back to your rooms to read, listen to music or lectures, or to entertain. No snacks were taken back to nibble on and there was no corner shop, from which to buy tempting but unhealthy morsels.

With the influx of Western Jewry from America, Britain and Europe, came bad eating habits; particularly the American habits of eating in the streets, using food as a solace, and overloading one's plate with too much food on almost every social occasion. So many Israeli social occasions seemed to revolve around food; hospitality was so generous that no one left the table before they felt uncomfortably full.

On the other hand Israel had developed the most modern hospitals and medical techniques and had excellent health screening programmes. The natural resources of the Dead Sea were already used to treat conditions such as psoriasis and arthritis. Advanced agricultural techniques produced a variety of newly developed fruits and vegetables. I just knew if there was a way to combine all these products and services while at the same time relieving some of the stress and tension of daily Israeli life, and changing the nation's poor eating habits, Israel could well become the health capital of the world. With medical costs so high in America and almost 30 million Europeans entitled to use their health insurance programmes in Israel, I saw a number of ways in which a new health industry could be developed.

One of the first projects I was involved with was the creation of a health resort on the Dead Sea; this was to be a joint venture involving a group of Born Again Christians (they believed in the Biblical prophecy that proclaimed the curative and healing powers of the Dead Sea). Our plan for turning that spa into the Twenty-First Century Health Enhancement and Disease Prevention Centre was delayed, but a spa is now open and the Dead Sea treatment centres have almost a hundred per cent year-round occupancy.

It was during that time that I began meeting 'healers', spiritualists and experts in nutritional programmes whose roots lay in the prophesies and stories of the Bible. It was an exciting time and I was thrilled by the open simplicity and fervour of these people. We began to develop together new health and diet foods which we hoped to export from Israel.

Not long after Richard's death I met a widower, a scientist called Lorenz Anschell. His wife had died some time before, after a long illness; like me he was emotionally wounded. We became good friends — just good friends.

Larry was opposed to tranquillizing medication of any kind, and with his help I continued the fight to free myself of this dependency. I remembered how helpful exercise had been in the past and I also began to substitute natural and alternative remedies. I found myself visiting health food shops searching for exotic biblical and herbal remedies. It seemed to me that some of the prepared foods found in these shops were far from healthy. Additives and preservatives were not used in line with current trends, but many of the products were kept on display long after their shelf life. I saw besides that many of the foods which were sought after by people on diets contained ingredients that were actually very fattening.

By the mid 1980s there was a growing interest in weight reducing programmes which involved prepared diet foods. I knew of the earlier, very low-calorie diets — VLCDs as they were called — and they worried me. I was concerned about people consuming only 330 calories while pursuing a normal active day. I was even more concerned about the way in which these VLCDs were being sold. The selling procedures amounted to a form of legalized 'pyramid selling' now called direct marketing. Untrained people anxious to earn money quickly were selling large quantitites of these products without any medical supervision. I was outraged to discover that a 16-year-old anorexic had been able to purchase a three months' supply from a part-time secretary who sold to her without question.

I realized, however, that direct selling was becoming popular and was delighted to learn that an alternative direct selling approach was being introduced in the USA to sell a complete programme of behaviour modification, exercise and an 800—1,000 calories per day diet. The prepared foods were retort foods. These were created for the US astronaut programme and had been successfully tested. They had a shelf-life of two to five years, were easily transportable, and needed only the briefest heating to make them ready for eating. They were more than palatable, some of the samples I tasted were delicious, and they gave the dieter a wide range of choices.

One of the physicians with whom I had worked in Israel, Professor Charles Kleeman, now headed a programme at the University of Southern California which was preparing all the behaviour modification material and working with the University of Arizona which prepared audio tapes and video tapes to teach exercise. This seemed an extremely interesting programme and I was invited to the United States to meet the entrepreneurs who had started it.

I was interested to find that many of the people to whom they were addressing the programme were 'drop-outs' from the USA Cambridge Diet and Herbal Life Programmes as well as other Very Low Calorie Diet-type operations. It was an impressively put together administrative programme and the foods certainly were superior to powdered drinks.

During this time I became involved with a Canadian product called the Nutri Diet, and upon further investigation I discovered there was an American company called Nutri/Systems which was running weight-loss centres using prepared foods, computerized diets and a serious programme of behavioural modification; this company was growing quickly in the United States and rapidly becoming popular. I entered into negotiations with Nutri/Systems about the possibility of joining forces with them, but not before I had already invested large sums of money as well as vast amounts of time and energy in a programme to produce retort foods in Israel. I was also investigating retort food production in England, Scotland and Ireland.

With this new technology and the tremendous support and buying power of religions-oriented Christians and Jews who were seeking their roots once again in the Bible, I felt it would be interesting to create a programme marketing health and diet foods that were actually 'commanded to be eaten' or were the staples of our prophets and biblical heroes. In furtherance of this I prepared a new diet called, appropriately, 'The Jerusalem Diet'.

I entered into negotiations with the largest of Israel's companies. Koor was a major conglomerate by any terms. Its interests stretched into every aspect of the nation's life from defence, through foods, into the latest technology. It was very anxious to enter the health field and produce diet foods which could be exported widely.

By this time there was an expanding interest in such low-calorie eating programmes which sold ready-prepared meals. I thought of creating a regime using these foods as part of my Jerusalem Diet, particularly the seven varieties of food promised by God to Joshua: milk, honey, wheat, barley, grapes, dates and pomegranates.

Eventually I planned to offer a combination of four different, complementary approaches drawn together in what I decided to call WiseWeighs. This was a new company which I established to offer medically supervised weight-loss and fitness centres, with ready-made meals available for purchase by members at these centres. There would be behaviour modification classes run by trained psychologists, and counsellors would offer group therapy for motivation, suggesting ways of finding personal solutions to weight and weight-related problems. Because of the introduction of exercise as a serious component of this concept, I hoped to attract not only overweight people but people who were not fat but also not fit. These people would be interested in making exercise a regular part of their lifestyle but also anxious to learn about healthy eating habits. The fact that there would be medical assessments and medical supervision made me feel that the numerous direct selling operations which were flooding the market would have to 'pull their socks up' to compete with us and thus I was doing what I had done in the early days of Weight Watchers — being responsible for, and raising the standards of, my industry.

In the early summer of 1986 I was approached by Guinness, who had learned of my activities. Although the public tended to think of Guinness only in connection with brewing, the company had already spent millions of pounds since 1984 building up the nucleus of a healthcare business which they called the Portman Health Group. They had already acquired Gleneagles Hotel in Scotland and then added Champneys health spa in Tring, Cranks vegetarian restaurant chain, Nature's Best (a mail order vitamin firm), and another company, Dietary Specialities, which marketed natural vitamin supplements. Guinness originally contemplated purchasing Nutri/Systems but instead it was suggested to them that they should begin a joint venture with me to develop WiseWeighs which they believed was a more comprehensive approach than Nutri/ Systems. They made .me a most attractive offer which included all the obvious benefits that only a large company with substantial resources could offer — administrative assistance, offices, equipment, a wide range of specialists in real estate, marketing, advertizing, promotion, and the opportunities of combining the activities of WiseWeighs with those of their existing hotel, health spa and restaurants.

Although I had planned to keep Israel as my home base, things had changed considerably in my life. Larry, to whom I had grown close and with whom I contemplated a possible union, had earlier decided to move to Australia because of his work, and expected that I would marry him and settle there. I felt it wouldn't be fair to uproot Alesia again; I certainly wasn't prepared to leave her, or to add yet another continent to my life. Now that Richard was dead I wanted to be more available for the boys and strengthen family links. Instead of travelling every eight days to keep contact with the boys strong, I decided that England — where the children had been born and the boys had been educated — might be the best place to set up an office and a new base.

Guinness was anxious to finalize the deal with me, fearing I might join Nutri/Systems in its expansion into the UK. Despite the urgency created by their own deadlines, their offer and the terms of our contract changed many times before everything was finally signed. It was not a promising start, to say the least — but I was elated by the opportunity it offered.

During negotiations, I was told th Ernest Saunders, then chairman of Guinness, had seen the writing on the wall; public attitudes towards the consumption of alcohol were changing as growing numbers of people began to take health concerns seriously. I was assured that I could help take Guinness forward into the twenty-first century. Instead

I found myself going up a blind alley.

One of the difficulties was that no one in the Saunders-run company really understood what my business was about. Outside advisers recommended a further £5 million investment in the health care business and approved my business plan; they did not take into account that the real value of the business lay in the quality of its staff, the service we provided, and the products; no one even attempted to evaluate the possibilities of the new foods I was developing. They were dazzled by projections which were impressive but which meant little in themselves.

What was worse, Guinness found it difficult to fulfil many of the agreed conditions of our working relationship; the lessons I learned from that experience were both substantial and expensive.

WiseWeighs was the newest company to join the Portman Health Group and almost from the start I was made to feel that I was a burden rather than an asset. I had been promised office accommodation and staff but it was a battle to get either. One day I would have a typewriter and no secretary, the next I would have a secretary but no typewriter. It was no way to run a business. Guinness had its own problems consolidating the Distillers Company acquisition, and found it difficult to give me time or space. They probably forgot I was there some of the time.

My contract gave me control over the hiring of key officers and members of staff; each time I suggested someone as a managing director, there was always some reason why my choice was deemed inappropriate or a decision must be delayed indefinitely. David Smith, my first choice as adviser and acting managing director, was described by one of Guinness's executives as someone who would 'never amount to anything'. David, as chairman of Isoceles, subsequently captured all the business headlines by masterminding the largest takeover the city had ever experienced with a £2 billion takeover of Gateway Food-markets.

A good example of the way Guinness worked under Ernest Saunders was the story of the company car. It was decided that all executives in our subsidiary should be asked to take part in a three-day management seminar. We would be lectured and also take part in discussions about how to be creative, original and inventive in order to stay 'one step ahead'. The day after the seminar I was told that I was entitled to a company car worth a certain sum, in accordance with my status as chief executive and chairman of WiseWeighs. 'Your car will be a Volvo,' they said.

When I indicated that I wanted a Jaguar in the same price range as the Volvo, an argument ensued, which ended up with my being told that I could only have a Volvo. 'In any case,' said the Guinness executive dealing the matter, 'it will be impossible for you to buy a Jaguar, because there is a two-year waiting list. I'm so certain about it,' he continued, 'that if you do manage to get one, I will personally pay for it!' That night, on television, I saw an interview with a man who claimed he could immediately find any make of car for a potential purchaser. When I rang he wasn't there but his wife was and she turned out to have been one of my early Weight Watchers 50-pound losers. When I explained what I wanted, she said she would deal with it. That was Friday night. On Sunday her husband arrived with not one but two cars, from which I was to choose. On Monday morning when the man at the Guinness office saw my Jaguar, the colour drained from his face.

Being a lady, I didn't insist he keep his part of the bargain, but the episode illustrated the madness — and sadness — of the situation.

Earlier in that same year, Guinness was involved in a £2.7 billion battle with the Argyll Food Chain for control of the Distillers Drinks empire; a battle which ultimately led to seven leading city figures, including the former chairman of Guinness, Ernest Saunders, being convicted of fraud and other offences.

On December 1st 1986, three months after I began

working with Guinness, the Department of Trade and Industry announced they had begun an investigation into the takeover of the Distillers Company. After that it was bedlam. Everything I did — or tried to do — was blocked or queried endlessly by outside advisers or minor executives to whom I was 'handed over'. The headlines in the press were talking about missing millions, yet I was having to justify authorizing a £2.80 fare on my taxi account for one of my staff!

One of the lessons I learned from Weight Watchers was the importance of building up people's confidence and self-respect in order to get the best out of them. Demoralizing your staff, burying them in paperwork and making them feel inadequate or untrustworthy was counter-productive.

Much was written subsequently about the trial of the 'Gang of Four'. It lasted four months, to be followed by a second Guinness trial. Having first become acquainted with Ernest Saunders when he was both chairman and chief executive of Guinness, I would say that no trial in a court of law or even his sentence could equal the unbelievable pain and punishment that his fall from grace had already brought him. Although I was not an admirer of his style of management, I believe that he carried too great a share of the blame for what was happening generally in the financial world and particularly among the City of London's financial institutions.

That business world has become a jungle; here energetic, creative entrepreneurs are under constant risk of being swallowed up by highly experienced financial sharks, who swim through the sometimes muddy waters of the British takeover business, swallowing fine and substantial enterprises; they spit out 'bits' — fine companies which once were the source of great pride to the people who created them and gave excellent service to consumers, while employing a dedicated and honourable staff. These take-overs were frequently applauded by the public who seem to have traded in their favourite football heroes for these new takeover stars — the raiders and ruiners of small, middle-sized, as well as old established businesses in the UK.

Accepting the Guinness proposal meant another change for both Alesia and me. Whereas Israel would always be home to us both, running a company in England while my base remained Israel, involved considerable expense in terms of hotel accommodation in London, moving files, materials and an entire office block to England; worse still, my going back to work meant resettling Alesia in a 'dreaded boarding school'. Two marvellous friends, Franklin and Marcia Littell, recommended a Quaker school in Pennsylvania. The George School was to change all my views about boarding schools in general.

The Quaker attitude towards involvement in the community, responsibility for one's neighbours and for the world's problems and the concept of 'friends' and family made it an ideal place for Alesia, after the warm, emotional (but unstructured) society that Alesia had experienced during her schooling in Israel. Somehow these diverse philosophies of life blended well. Alesia was able to continue her dancing career with a marvellous group in Philadelphia and our friends Marciarose and Jerry Shestack became surrogate parents, providing a home, away from home, not only for Alesia but for Douglas, who was now at Princeton University and for Graeme, who was at the University of Pennsylvania in Philadelphia. Although our family home was in Israel and my office in England, in fact, 'home base' became Philadelphia, and the Shestacks and the Littells reintroduced us all to the warmth of American friendship as well as the wonders of America.

This meant, however, that England was a round of hotels and impersonal living for me, during my negotiations with Guinness and later while I was trying to set up the company. A fairy godmother appeared in the form of Dr Miriam Rothschild. We had met in Israel some years back. My first influential friend and mentor in England had been Sir John Foster, one of Nature's true gentlemen — larger than life when painted on any canvas. He helped me in the early days of Weight Watchers, and in the custody case. Miriam had been his closest friend and we met after his death to discuss a memorial for him. During the difficult custody trial concerning Alesia, Miriam had generously offered me her home, sound advice and warm and patient guidance. She represented all I admired in womanhood and reminded me greatly of my grandmother, possessing the same phenomenal energy and boundless interest in others. Her help and support in this difficult and challenging period of my life helped me immeasurably.

Guinness's problems with the Department of Trade and Industry intensified. Soon a new management team was brought in. They saw, quite rightly, that Guinness had to consolidate. The Portman Health Division, however worthwhile, was a departure from the group's main sphere of operations in the food and drink industry.

I was sympathetically treated by the new Chairman, and particularly by one board member, Brian Baldock, a man I admired and whose career I had followed with great interest since early days when he was a fan of Weight Watchers. Through the good offices of Lord Lever we negotiated WiseWeighs' amicable separation from the Guinness company. I was happy to work with them again recently during British-Soviet Month in Moscow — and would have been happier still had I bought shares in this now splendidly managed company.

My business association with Guinness left my confidence shaken, however, and I mourned the time lost and the products and foods which I had helped to pioneer. Many of these can now be found on the shelves of major British food shops.

After the Guinness settlement I returned to Israel. While I was there I received an invitation to visit the Soviet Union. I was told that the Ministry of Health there wished to discuss with me the use of group therapy and some of my more recent behaviour modification techniques and perhaps use these in their treatment of drug and alcohol addiction as well as the treatment of obesity. Apparently, during a visit to England, Mrs Gorbachev had seen a programme or read an article about me and my work with Weight Watchers. I was told she had a daughter who was interested in the behavioural approach to the treatment of drug addiction and alcohol abuse; she hoped that I might be able to share some of my expertise.

In December 1987 I set off with seven suitcases loaded with WiseWeighs foods, books, examples of our dietary and exercise programme, and material which I had produced in Israel, Switzerland and the UK contained in video tapes, audio tapes, and many cartoons and illustrations.

I also took with me a list of twenty Soviet-Jewish families — Refuseniks, who were desperately trying to leave the Soviet Union and settle in Israel. I remained in the Soviet Union for almost three weeks. Nothing that I had read or seen prepared me for the complete shock I felt during that first visit. My parents had told me about the Russia they chose to remember — through songs, exciting and joyous dances, and folk tales. What I found was morose, unhappy, unhealthy-looking people, many wandering the streets quite intoxicated, even early in the day. It was the shabbiness and sense of loss that I saw in the faces of men, women and children — particularly in Moscow — that upset me most. Because of the shortages, particularly the lack of fresh fruit and vegetables, the food offered in restaurants was limited and for the most part greasy, overcooked and without taste. I could well understand why alcoholism might be an attractive alternative.

I was also concerned to find that many of the younger women who were now finding it easier to obtain fashion magazines from England, America, France and Germany, were becoming obsessed with slimness and dieting; anorexia and bulimia were now growing problems in the Soviet Union.

I visited several hospitals and the Institute of Nutrition,

and met with the Director of the Temperance Society, who claimed he had 40 million active members. It became clear that whereas there were a growing number of Russians suffering from a variety of eating disorders, most of the treatments available in the Soviet Union for obesity were ineffective and costly. Some of the methods of treatment made my hair stand on end. They were even worse than the earlier experimentation in this country when patients' jaws were wired or radical bypass surgery and intravenous feeding were first attempted.

There was no information given to overweight patients about nutrition, even after their treatments; they simply became fat once again. Anorexics were threatened with incarceration in asylums and no one knew how to treat bulimics. It was not that the medical profession was uncaring but that they had neither the manpower nor the resources to provide alternative treatments.

My recommendation of group therapy as a simple alternative was warmly welcomed and the two model centres we set up began to work quickly and well. When I told them the case histories of people like Jean Renwick and Dolly Wager, who were helped only by the interaction of lay groups working alongside the medical profession, both doctors and government officials were impressed. I prepared a 12-week initial programme which these groups started to implement. I suggested that in addition to the material that I had left with them on nutrition and behaviour modification techniques, they use some of their own information on exercise, garnered from the training which had brought to the world's attention some of the finest Russian and Eastern European gymnasts and sportsmen.

Having visited the new microsurgery hospital created by Professor Fyodorov, I knew that under proper direction, and with inspired personal and creative energy, obesity could be reduced and prevented cheaply and just as effectively as Russian scientists were addressing other medical problems.

From what I have been told, the two groups I helped to

start have been an unqualified success. I understand that the original classes have now expanded to 16 and *TASS* has reported that 600 women's groups have now requested the opportunity of running weight control classes.

While I was in Moscow I was invited to attend a state occasion with some physicians I had met. Suddenly the group with whom I was talking, stiffened and appeared surprised. I turned around to see Mrs Gorbachev coming towards us. She had an interpreter with her, but in fact she did speak English. After a few pleasantries she asked if I was comfortable and whether there was anything that she could do for me. 'Yes,' I said, taking a list of the twenty Refusenik families out of my handbag, 'I have here the case histories of Jewish families in deep distress whose stories I would like to acquaint you with. I wonder if you would grant me the favour of looking into their case histories.'

Her face turned brick red and I could see she was very angry. She said, 'I thought you were a clever woman.' I replied, 'I am.' She then asked why I would risk raising such a sensitive subject at such an early stage in our relationship. I explained that my parents had left the Soviet Union in search of religious freedom and I, who had grown up in the United States, had benefitted from that freedom; I was deeply sympathetic towards people who were not so fortunate. I added, politely but firmly, that although I had been invited to the Soviet Union as a guest, I had made a point of financing all the programmes I started myself; I pointed out that if anyone was indebted to anyone it was the Soviet Union that was now indebted to me, rather than the other way round. I also pointed out that I was particularly moved by the cases of the women, many of whom had been advised that the best way out of Russia was to divorce their husbands and leave with their children for Israel. Later, their men might be allowed to follow. In fact, in many instances, these families had been separated for as long as eighteen years, the husbands still petitioning for permission to leave for Israel.

Lastly I said, perhaps cheekily, that my father had taught me in Brooklyn that if someone offers, you should take. Since she had made such a generous offer, I had decided to take her at her word.

She said nothing for what seemed like hours; everyone around us began to shift their feet and look away in embarrassment. I, too, began to feel uncomfortable and dropped my head. She poked me firmly in the shoulder and said, 'I will see your list.' She suggested that I hand the papers to an aide — they would go through the proper channels — but she would 'investigate'.

Since that time I have had the privilege and honour of welcoming many of those people whose names were on my list when they arrived in Israel. I was later overjoyed to take part in a ceremony with many of these Refuseniks when we honoured the Prime Minister of Australia, Bob Hawke, for his unflinching championship of their cause, and am still in touch with many of the families whose emigration from Russia I — in common with many human rights advocates, Jewish and non-Jewish — helped to secure.

But that night in particular, as I left the unbelievably impressive and beautiful walls of the Kremlin, I felt a special sense of pleasure. I knew Momma and Poppa, and particularly my grandmother, would have been pleased with me.

CHAPTER TEN

'Thou art weighed in the balance and art found wanting'

Book of Daniel, V, vii

During the time I was in Russia I learned that my friend Larry faced serious health problems. I left for Australia to be with him. While he was in hospital after surgery I spent long hours over many months talking with him. As a scientist he was appalled at what he considered the unstructured manner in which I had lived my life since I left Weight Watchers, misdirecting my energies and not caring for myself emotionally or physically. As a professor and a physicist he was inquisitive, exacting and directive and wanted me to think and to plan logically each step in my life and towards my next career.

I was, he said, one of the people who made things happen in life, but he wanted to lead me into a new pattern of thinking, a determination that intensified when he knew he was going to die. This new resource towards which he was guiding me was to be his last gift to me, a preparation for a new kind of life in which I would be better able to preserve both my health and material resources.

Sitting around the hospital and eating carelessly, I felt flabby, strained and out of shape. I began to cycle and to work out with a trainer who took me for long walks on Bondi Beach. After Larry's death I found myself generally more aware, studying more carefully the effect that my long walks on Bondi Beach had on burning up the calories I was consuming. I expanded my activities into cycling, brisk walking, stair climbing, swimming and light weight-training. Later, when visiting health hydros, exercise camps and health resorts, I added Tai Chi and even went back to the games of my youth in Brooklyn — basketball and volleyball. This time I found myself working with stop-watches and pedometers and doing mental and written sums calculating the calories I was burning and the improvement these exercises were having on my metabolic rate.

It would have been very hard, if not impossible, to exercise on my own. Grief has a way of turning one inward. Larry's boys and my new friends provided me with a surrogate group, similar to the group therapy of Weight Watchers in the past. This, combined with the healing qualities of Australia's majestic land, made Alice Springs, Ayers Rock, the Gold Coast and rain forests peerless gymnasiums in which to do my 'walkabouts'. I resolved to take charge of my own health and happiness in a disciplined and logical way, in tribute to Larry and all those who had helped me. I began to think deeply about where I was and where I had been.

When you devote your life to something, part of the reward of doing so is that your chosen subject's subtleties and complexities reveal themselves to you — not immediately but in stages, over time, like so many layers of an onion. It isn't easy to stick with — maybe that's why an onion makes you cry — but it can mean the difference in your degree of understanding.

Since the age of 11, the problems of weight and health have been my obsession, and to them I have devoted my entire adult life. Today, I sit on top of a mountain of information and understanding about weight loss; a mountain that is always growing, as knowledge comes gradually. It started, as it had to, by my being fat and consequently unhappy. This led serendipitously to Weight Watchers and to tremendous success. To this day, when I hear of yet another successful step forward by what was my baby (now an upright 24-year-old), I react with motherly pride and delight.

But as one grows, one learns, and certainly I am no different. From Weight Watchers and England, to Switzerland and Slim-Fit, to Israel and the original WiseWeighs, to

Australia and my new appreciation of exercise — I have gleaned and collected my stories of Weight Wisdom so that what I now impart to you in this final section of the book is a 'how-to' based on my own life. My problems and my need for solutions over the years are not peculiar to me, but are shared by millions. Despite the phenomenal growth in the health food, fad diet and gym markets, unhappily these problems persist. It is time for us take another layer off the onion.

One of the most important things I have learned about the principles of dieting and weight loss was foreshadowed during my very early days at Weight Watchers. During the initial stages of the development of the company in England, I was told by a leading psychiatrist that I was not in the weight business at all. 'You are involved with transitional energy,' said Dr Harold Bridger, Head of the Tavistock Clinic for Organizational Change and advisor to many major companies on business dynamics and interpersonal work relations. 'What your lecturers do with that energy will spell their future success or failure,' he continued.

Dr Bridger was referring to the energy which Weight Watchers men and women created by change — or, more importantly, by the *feeling* of change. As they lost weight, they felt re-born. Suddenly, they were able to experience an exhilaration derived from being totally different. This in turn created energy acting as a catalyst to reinforce that difference.

At that time, I didn't grasp the full impact of Dr Bridger's insight. The average age of a Weight Watcher's member was 45. I was then in my early thirties and although I could sympathize with and comprehend my members' concerns and trials, I hadn't personally experienced the whole spectrum of them.

In Australia in 1988, alone and in danger of stagnating, I realized I needed literally to get moving. I began to think about the many women I had met on my journeys and the many conversations I had had with Weight Watchers members who confided in me how hard it was to begin any new regime — and stick to it. Exercise or movement was often just too much to contemplate during times of crisis or emotional stress. I also realized how little overweight people moved at all in their normal lives and how this physical immobility sometimes resulted in mental immobility as well.

This was when the full force of Harold Bridger's transitional energy theory merged with Dr George Sheehan's credo in his seminal work *Sheehan on Running* in which he explained how he had pulled the emergency cord on the inactivity which was heading him on the road to premature death or ill health — and began to run for his life. Only I had to walk before I ran.

I resolved to take all I had learned from Weight Watchers, all I had absorbed from synectics and the New Age movement, and all I had experienced using exercise both as a stimulant and an added dimension in controlling weight. I had learned also that in moments of trial, crisis or transition, to move mountains one must first *move oneself.*

Thus was WiseWeighs re-born. (For a fuller explanation of its aims and achievements see the next chapter). Central to its philosophy is a concept which I have developed into an exercise-based diet which anyone can follow: I call it the Bank Balance Diet, but it is more than a diet, much more.

The Bank Balance Diet provides the key to establishing a way of life — a regime for living — which will promote an attractive weight and maintain good health. I have set it out more fully in a book called *The Bank Balance Diet,* sub-titled 'an investment programme that puts your health into credit for life while making you look and feel like a millionaire'.

The basic principle behind the Bank Balance Diet is that weight and health, like money, have to be managed carefully and constantly. Managing our money is a basic fact of our lives, balancing what we have against what we can afford. Managing our weight and health is a matter of putting in and taking out calories in much the same way, so that at the end of the day we are not overdrawn.

So the Bank Balance Diet is based on the idea of regarding eating and exercise as debits and credits on a current account. The more you put into your account in terms of exercise, the more you can take out in terms of eating what you like — and still lose weight, or remain slim.

The Bank Balance Diet is the 'thinking person's diet' — and it does require thought because it involves making choices. Essentially, the question you ask yourself is, 'How far would I walk for a Mars bar?'

Nothing is forbidden, but in order to have the foods you desire, you must know what they will 'cost' you in terms of calories, and how much credit you need to have in terms of exercise to be able to afford them. After a while these calculations become second nature.

In the Bank Balance Diet *you* are the banker and that's a mighty powerful person to be. Remember when you played Monopoly as a child, the special joy of being the banker in the game? Handing out the properties and the money gave you a tremendous sense of importance and a feeling that you had the edge on everyone else. Similarly, being your own banker when you follow the Bank Balance Diet can give you those same feelings of power and security.

It works like this: you earn credit through exercise and use up some of that credit every time you eat. Your bank opens in the morning when you wake — when you eat something it's akin to writing a cheque or using your credit card; unless you have sufficient funds in your account you go into the red. You will pay for mismanagement of your diet banking account by putting on weight, unless you do some exercise.

You can think of meal times as your standing orders. You know that a certain amount will be deducted from your account at a particular point in time. You also know that you should make certain there will be enough funds in your account to cover this.

Those funds are created by exercise — the sport, the walking, the movement, the activity — you have taken and have calculated will cover your withdrawals. Ideally, if you wish to lose weight, you should stay permanently in credit through exercise.

To be able to balance your account, you need to know the exact calorific content of different foods. In Weight

Watchers, although we knew the calorific content of the basic Programme, we never discussed this because we felt people ate food not calories. That still makes good sense. However, once you introduce an exercise element into any eating programme you need to know how many calories there are in, for instance, a slice of cake in order to know what you have to do in terms of exercise to 'earn' it. In order to follow the Bank Balance Diet you need to have an idea of the calorific content of the foods you like and which can be combined in a healthy balanced diet.

My forthcoming book *The Bank Balance Diet* will provide a guide to calories taken in as food plus how much 'credit' doing certain exercises or movements will give you in burning calories off. It should prove an invaluable aid to balancing your personal diet books.

BUILDING UP THE DEBITS AND CREDITS OF YOUR DIET BANK BALANCE

Your body needs a basic number of calories each day just to keep you sleeping, talking and fulfilling your normal daily activities. This is your normal bank balance or your basic metabolic rate (BMR). If you eat more calories than your body can use, the extra calories will be stored as fat and you will gain weight.

TOO MANY CALORIES WILL PUT YOU IN DEBIT

If you consume fewer calories than your body needs (either by eating less or through exercise), your body will look to its own fuel stores for energy. It will burn the fat and carbohydrates already stored and you will lose weight.

USING UP CALORIES SO THAT YOU GO BELOW YOUR DAILY BANK BALANCE WILL PUT YOU IN CREDIT

You will be a happy diet bank manager and your body will be a satisfied customer.

If you continue so that you have a 3,500 calorie credit then you will have lost — or paid off to the bank — one pound of fat. Remember that key fact: 3,500 calories equals one pound.

There are several considerations regarding diet and exercise which affect the way your body loses or gains weight. To understand these, and to implement my Bank Balance Diet, first you must understand the way your body operates.

YOUR METABOLISM

By definition your metabolism is those chemical and physical processes in your body which provide energy so that your body can function. Your body gets exercise from calories obtained from food. You may have heard someone mention that they have a 'fast' or a 'slow' metabolism. One with a fast metabolism will burn more calories than will someone with a slow metabolism. The faster (or more efficient) your metabolism becomes, the easier you will lose weight. In Bank Balance Diet terms, a person with a fast metabolism might be said to have a low interest rate on their normal bank balance — that is, they won't gain weight as easily as someone with a higher interest rate.

Because regular exercise increases your metabolism, it will add to the number of calories you burn and increase your ability to lose weight. But exercise not only burns more calories when you are actually moving, it also keeps your metabolism up for several hours after you finish. When comparing two people of the same size, the person who is fit will use more calories sleeping than the less fit one.

Muscle cells are more active and therefore use more calories than fat cells. Therefore, a person with more muscle (for example, a man) actually has a higher metabolism than a person of the same height and weight with less muscle (a woman). Since exercise increases your muscle mass, exercise will speed up your metabolism! As an aid to a higher metabolism and keeping your bank balance in credit so that you will lose weight, exercise and increased muscle mass are crucial.

FAT AND CARBOHYDRATES

To be more specific, your metabolism is fuelled by the food calories you eat. It is very important to be aware that not all calories are equal. Some calories are more fattening than others. Note: 100 calories of chocolate are more fattening than 100 calories of a banana. Here's why.

The fibre in a banana slows the absorption of the calories, so they are less likely to trigger the release of insulin which stores calories unused at the time. The carbohydrate and fat in chocolate raises the blood levels of sugar quickly, and trigger the release of insulin so that the body stores more of the calories as fat.

EXCHANGE RATE MECHANISM

There are three types of calories from which you get your energy: fat, carbohydrate and protein. It is important to remember that they are more or less interchangeable in the body, energy-wise. Because protein is used mainly to build the tissues, like nails, hair, and skin, it is used only as energy in severe cases of starvation (such as anorexia nervosa). Therefore fat and carbohydrates are the main energy sources for our body.

One could think of them as three currencies which can be exchanged. The actual rates of exchange are carbohydrate, 4 calories per gram, protein 9 calories per gram and fat 9 calories per gram.

When we eat carbohydrates our body uses them almost immediately for quick energy. When we eat fat, it is stored in the body and only used later. For this reason (unless one is a lumberjack), it is better to eat a high carbohydrate diet. It is only when one eats *too many* carbohydrates that they will be stored as fat. Excess protein is also stored in the body as fat, which is why high protein diets are often not recommended.

HOW TO BURN FAT

When we need a sudden or powerful burst of energy it will be obtained from the carbohydrate (or glycogen) stores in our muscles. If we were to continue this movement for an extended period of time, the body would sense that it is very uneconomical to keep using carbohydrates as the main fuel source. We have a limited supply of carbohydrates which must be replenished by eating. Fat, on the other hand, is abundant throughout the body even on a 'skinny' person. After about 15 minutes or so the body realizes that continuing at its current rate of anaerobic activity (burning carbohydrates for fuel), it will eventually run out and the body will become fatigued, so it switches over to the more efficient aerobic metabolism which uses fat for fuel. Fat will be used from all over the body including the face, arms, torso, hips and legs.

The body's metabolic system works much like a car. When it first starts moving it shifts into first gear, and as it increases speed and power it shifts into second. These are the anaerobic phases of energy providing and carbohydrates are used for fuel. Soon the body realizes it will deplete its fuel if it does not economize, so it starts using a higher percentage of fat. In this gear it can survive for a very long period of time (hence the endurance of a marathon runner or other aerobic athletes).

So when you want to lose body fat, scientists recommend that you do aerobic rather than anaerobic exercise. Often anaerobic exercises (sprinting, weight lifting, sit-ups and other floor exercises) use up only the carbohydrates and have water as a by-product. This is why people can sweat and lose water when dieting, easily regaining the pounds lost (as water and fat) when they drink again.

The best type of credit to add to your bank balance is one

from low-impact aerobic exercise such as walking, cycling, running, stair-climbing, dancing, swimming and such types of exercise. This type of debit will actually decrease your fat and change your body shape through the loss of unsightly inches from fat-deposit areas such as the abdomen, hips and thighs. So if your goal is to have a flatter stomach, it is more effective to walk for 30 minutes and burn the fat off rather than to do hundreds of stomach exercises which will utilize only carbohydrates, and strengthen the muscle without eliminating the fat surrounding it.

YOUR BODY COMPOSITION: MUSCLE VS FAT

Another important aspect to consider is your own body composition. This is the make-up of your body between lean body mass and fat. Lean body mass includes muscles, bones, nervous tissue, skin and organs. It is the active part of your body — the part that uses energy. Fat represents stored energy. Although a minimum amount of fat is essential for protection of the vital organs, excess fat can cause a variety of ailments including heart diseases and diabetes.

Fat is also responsible for the way your body looks. Therefore, when dieting, it is more sensible to try to decrease body fat measured through the loss of inches rather than to try to lose pounds (which could constitute vital body fluids and muscle tissue). You can measure your own body fat in several ways; the most accurate is the underwater tank test, the more accessible is the skin caliper which gives a very lose estimate of your actual figure. Most health clubs offer this testing service. At home you could measure your fat/weight loss through inches rather than pounds.

WHY DIET ALONE IS NOT THE BEST WAY
TO LOSE FAT

Studies have shown that the best way to lose body fat is through a combination of aerobic (fat-burning) exercise such as walking and a reduced-calorie diet with an emphasis on eating less fatty foods and more carbohydrates. Exercise alone will help reduce body fat, but dieting alone is not recommended for several reasons which will be discussed later.

When people diet, they consume less than the minimum amount of calories the body needs for energy each day. In other words, they eat less food than the body metabolism needs to operate. As a result the body uses the stored energy that is available.

If one reduces calorie intake too much (such as on a very low-calorie diet), the body will react in a defensive way and lower its BMR or minimum number of calories needed each day. Once very low-calorie dieters return to their normal eating habits they may actually gain weight since their metabolism is now lower. If they diet again and again, they may reduce their metabolic rate even more.

For example, if Jane normally needs about 2,000 calories a day just to walk, talk, sleep and so on, and she goes on a very low-calorie diet of 800 calories per day, her body may react by lowering its metabolic rate to requiring only 1,500 calories per day. In effect, the body slows down. When she returns to normal eating patterns of consuming, say, 1,800 calories a day she will actually *gain* weight. Prior to her diet she would have lost or at least maintained her weight, but now that her body has slowed she gains eating less than she could have before.

When a woman tries diet after diet, and keeps losing and gaining over a period of years, it is easy to see why a dieting method only is ineffective.

Very low-caloried diets are also dangerous from the nutritional standpoint. The fewer foods one eats, the fewer vitamins, minerals, proteins and carbohydrates one will consume. It is likely that one could become nutrient-deficient and suffer unhealthy side-effects as a result.

Along with a lower calorie-burning metabolic rate and nutrient deficit, very low-calorie diets can cause one to lose not only fat, but crucial muscle mass and body fluid. The body can actually degenerate from severe dieting.

The way one avoids the yo-yo effect and keeps the metabolism high is by including fat-burning aerobic exercise in the weight-loss programme.

THE BANK BALANCE DIET EXPLAINED

The wonderful thing about the Bank Balance Diet is that it is your own personalized bank which you alone manage. You, not a prescribed diet plan, choose what you eat and what you do. It's very simple and there is freedom to tailor the process to fit your individual requirements and preferences.

As you can see, weight control is just a simple balance in the calories you eat and use. If you want to plan to lose 5 pounds of fat remember that a pound of fat is worth 3,500 calories. In order to lose 5 pounds you must then create a deficit of 17,500 calories in your diet. We recommend that you do it gradually, one day at a time.

You can create this deficit in several ways through a decreased calorie diet and an increase in daily exercise. Since walking briskly uses about 400 calories an hour if you walked an hour every day of the week for two weeks, you would use up 7,200 calories through exercise. That would leave you with only 10,300 calories to lose over a period of time. If you ate 500 calories less a day for two weeks (the equivalent to two small bars of chocolate) you would lose another 7,000 calories. At this point you would have already lost 4 pounds of fat (not muscle or water). You could safely assume that this is permanent weight loss and not temporary such as when you lose many pounds of water but regain it the minute you drink again. If you want to lose more weight all you have to do is exercise more and/or limit your calories (but not too much, so that you are still getting an adequate amount of nutrients).

People often ask when they should exercise and my answer is *whenever*. The hour doesn't matter so long as it is convenient to you. You can exercise when you wake, before or after a meal. Personally, however, I feel that if there must be a choice, exercise is best taken *before* meal times and definitely in the early morning before breakfast. This puts you in credit straight away, because not only will it re-open your account by stimulating your metabolic rate, which has lain fallow during the night, but you start the day by burning up calories.

One of the advantages of taking extra exercise early in the day or early in the week is that you can build up reserves through careful hoarding and this will give you an allowance you can splurge when you feel you need to. I would certainly recommend this approach, rather than one in which you plunge deeply into the red and then have to work like mad to clear your overdraft. Making sure you always have something in reserve is wise financial management. Just as Mr Micawber said: 'Annual income twenty pounds, annual expenditure nineteen pounds, nineteen shillings and sixpence — result, happiness. Annual income twenty pounds, annual expenditure twenty pounds and six pence — result, misery.' It is only a few pence each way, but those few pence add up to pounds.

Tests carried out at an aerobics centre in South Carolina indicate that people who exercise before a meal show a greater rate of weight loss and a more controlled maintenance than people who do not exercise before eating. It is not true that exercise works up an appetite; psychologically it reduces your appetite because you feel good about yourself and do not wish to spoil the effort you have made. Most truly fat people eat as a compensation for feeling bad, or to punish themselves further for something they have done wrong.

I would suggest that you start the day by walking; walking gives one time to think in the way that high-impact aerobics, for example, doesn't. An early morning walk is a wonderful opportunity to decide what healthy food you will eat moderately for breakfast.

Every day you will need to carry out an audit, to check the state of your account and do some future planning — the evening may seem the best time. However, in the evening it is tempting to take too expansive a view of your financial management and you may find a morning walk gives you the opportunity of being rather more ruthless.

You need to think about what the day has in store; when will you be hitting the low spots; what external cues will you encounter which may suddenly stimulate your appetite?

External cues are things which trigger your attention and consequently your consumption of food. A good example of this was shown by the behaviour of the pilots of Air France. Fat pilots had no problem flying into America and eating breakfast just after they had dinner on the plane. This was because the clock said it was breakfast time and they could see other people eating; these were the external cues. The thin pilots, on the other hand, had difficulty adjusting to the differences in meal times because they were not affected by the same external cues.

I also believe there are no set rules. If you choose to exercise after a meal this choice may help you to be more cautious about what you eat since you know you will have to burn it off afterwards. If you really are not looking forward to a lot of exercise, that will limit the amounts you eat. Instead of devouring an entire banana, for instance, you find yourself slicing half a banana very thinly and satisfying yourself with that. Or when you are putting low-fat spread on your toast and you are tempted to add jam or marmalade, you will resist because you know those extra calories will have to be worked off.

The important thing to remember about exercise is that it can help you increase your metabolic rate which is dependent on how much lean muscle tissue to fat you have in your body make-up. If through exercise you change the composition of your body by increasing the amount of lean muscle relative to fat, your metabolic rate will be increased, and you may eat more than you did before to stay the same weight without gaining.

Remember, the Bank Balance Diet puts *you* in control — gives you the power and the responsibility of literally shaping your new future as a slender and healthy individual.

CHAPTER ELEVEN

One of the things I've learned over the years is that although people are capable of enormous psychological adjustments and have the ability to change very radically, both for positive and negative reasons, there are certain social predelictions we have, or environments in which we perform best and seem happiest.

I believe in groups, and as a confirmed groupie tested the Bank Balance Diet with a control group in Ashton, near Oundle in Northamptonshire in my new WiseWeighs centre. Following the success of that scheme, there are now plans to open other centres.

WiseWeighs operates as a commercial organization which uses a group therapeutic approach to bring about weight loss. It promotes healthy behavioural and nutritional habits, and teaches the use of regular exercise as a way of promoting good health and fitness. It also provides, where possible, specially prepared foods for inclusion in a healthy, well-balanced slimming regime.

WiseWeighs centres aim to attract two types of people — the first is the overweight person who seeks a diet or dietary advice together with the group therapy support which has been fostered by organizations like Weight Watchers and other slimming groups. (Our groups will be run by qualified therapists.) The vast majority of these people are those who have either never exercised, have stopped exercising or who abhor exercise; they seek a comfortable protected environment in which to learn how to do normal exercise which will fit into the regular course of their daily lives.

WiseWeighs provides simple but adequate facilities which give members the opportunity to do basic stretching exercises, using chairs and stairs, and simple low-impact aerobic exercises. WiseWeighs also provides uncomplicated exercise machinery which enables people to feel they are in a health club environment.

The second group of people in WiseWeighs classes are those who are not fat but who are not fit. They approach WiseWeighs through exercise, but are as anxious to learn sensible nutrition and wish to be able to purchase our foods which are both healthy and dietetic, and also to discover behaviour modification techniques which will teach them good eating and exercise habits.

I believe that the best kind of exercise is the kind that can be done in all climates and in all weathers, and does not require special equipment or a special environment. Stair-climbing is one good example: everyone has at least one step in the house. I have also developed what I call chairobics; these too are ideal — everyone has a chair.

Stairobics and chairobics were some of the exercises we used in the pilot scheme. Our eldest member, Ginny Levin, was 82 and doing high kicks that would do justice to a Bluebell Girl. Our youngest, Rosemarie Minton, is now teaching regular exercises as a trained YMCA instructor — conducting classes for the elderly as well as people who haven't moved for years. In 8 weeks one member has lost 1st 12lb — her figure became as good as those she produces as a bookkeeper in Peterborough and Cambridge; even my housekeeper, Margaret Mears, tears around on her bike to do chores in Oundle — after years of physical inactivity.

The changes in us, the transition which this new group experienced, reminded me once again of all the other groups (mostly of women) I had worked with during my many-faceted career.

It seemed to me that their problems, caused by tran-sitional change or by other crises in their lives, could be resolved or at least improved with the assistance and healing powers of group support. Therefore out of Wise-Weighs I have developed a further concept, 'Women In Transition', or the WIT of WiseWeighs.

One of the things that fascinated me during the Weight Watcher years was the type of people who had been thin all their lives and then, without warning, suddenly began to put on weight. The weight they gained was in some instances very substantial and the weight gain was reasonably fast. Suddenly becoming fat was particularly trying to this group who had never had to worry about their weight or watch what they ate.

In analysing their problems we discovered that something major had happened to change their lives; some important transition.

With some it might have been a change of job or even getting married. Marriage may have taken them away from the group of friends with whom they formerly played a sport and consequently their regular exercise pattern was sharply altered. Many began to spend more time sitting behind a desk, driving a car or developing a social life which meant quiet evenings at home or a round of dinner parties with other newlyweds. Businessmen may have found that travel, entertaining clients or being abroad for long or short periods alone encouraged them to develop irregular eating patterns, to go on sudden splurges, to drink more heavily than usual.

Often for others, women, for example, these changes occurred after childbirth when they might feel the boredom of being at home with a small baby. A loss of job, too, might bring a loss of self-esteem. Another crisis point was often the menopause. Frequently it wasn't the hormonal changes themselves which were to blame, but the teaching of mothers and grandmothers who had said that the menopause automatically signalled weight gain. So the pattern was set.

Women often gained weight after a divorce. They felt less

attractive and their self-image was damaged. Again, after a bereavement, or when their children married and left home, many women felt their value to someone else, and thus to themselves, was diminished. They didn't count any more. My experience with Weight Watchers taught me that many women who were not fat from their early childhood, or in their teens, put on weight during times when they were in crisis. Alternatively, a minor weight problem became a major weight problem during crisis periods.

It was listening to these people that enabled me to understand that the group therapy we provided for Weight Watchers could also be helpful for people during transitional crises. By putting their problems into words, discussing them openly in a group, listening to suggestions, they could get their priorities straight and see the way forward. They could also seek professional advice in a form that was comfortable and socially acceptable to them.

One example of the kind of person who would benefit from our kind of help would be a woman recently bereaved. Her husband was the one who managed all the finances and made all major decisions in the family; now she is left as the principle provider, the economic regulator, and the person responsible for all the social, psychological and other needs of the family — including her children.

Such a woman would automatically be faced with a great number of problems all at once, at a time when she was weakened emotionally and psychologically and when her judgement might be questionable. Let us suppose, for example, the mortgage on the family house had been taken out a long time ago. Now she is suddenly the recipient of a substantial sum of money paid out by the insurance company on her husband's death. She is confused about how to invest the money, and unsure how to handle the mortgage repayments. Some well-meaning relative may advise her to use the lump sum to pay off the mortgage; this might have been fixed at 8 per cent, whereas invested, the money would have earned 15 per cent. In addition, she now finds herself saddled with a huge house which was ideal when she was a married woman in a social environment perfect for a couple, but where she now feels miserable as a single parent who must seek out the single life. She is in the wrong place and has now limited her opportunities to take holidays or do other things.

What she needs is an opportunity to determine what her main priority is. Usually, it is getting herself straight. Once she is straight and likes herself better, she is probably better able to deal with her children's and other family problems and certainly more capable of getting the advice and information she needs to make her decisions wisely. It is the WIT of WiseWeighs which will put her in a situation where she can say: 'These are the topics we want to discuss. I have been through a divorce, the loss of a husband or lover, and now I am on my own with certain responsibilities: what do I do first? Where do I get professional guidance?'

In my experience the woman wants to do something *dramatic* to herself — like losing weight — which will make her look different and pull her out of the rut. At the same time, she has to deal with practical problems. She may wish to get a job. A job today for the average woman means an understanding of computers and modern office equipment. To go to a computer class with 18-year-olds is looking for trouble and is likely to cause a further breakdown in her confidence. Instead she needs to find information about the kind of job that will be best suited for her, what skills she needs to bring to it, how to obtain those skills in a protected environment, what work she can manage if she has young children at home.

This is where WiseWeighs, having delineated what her priorities are, and having been able to point out what she must tackle first, can then help provide the expert advice she needs and the guidance to support her. The group is able to give her not only help with her weight problem but the chance to voice her wider fears and doubts, to help her sort out her priorities, and then give her the strength and support to help her deal with them.

Most of the people in my pilot scheme felt comfortable in a group with its emphasis on positive mental attitude — the group made them feel good about themselves and in no way reduced their sense of individuality. On the contrary, it enhanced and reinforced their sense of self-esteem.

For me, returning to a group after many years of being on my own was like coming home. For the first time I truly appreciated just how much the group element of Weight Watchers had meant to me and what a void my abrupt severance from the organization had caused in my life.

The years since Weight Watchers had been far from wasted though. I was able to bring to WiseWeighs not only the group concept pioneered by Weight Watchers but the benefits of my new research into nutrition, health, fitness, and hopefully the total well-being which the WIT of Wise-Weighs will promote.

In devizing the Bank Balance Diet and the WIT of WiseWeighs I have put myself back into the atmosphere of my happiest days as part of a warm community of people similarly motivated. It has caused the sparkle to return to my life, given me new direction and a sense of self-worth.

Writing my autobiography and telling the inspiring story of British Weight Watchers re-opened the doors to many of the rooms in my life I thought had been bolted and barred forever. Inside these rooms I found a wealth of memories. Some brought back old wounds, old pains — and sometimes these hurt badly; others revealed joys I had almost forgotten. That surprised me, but I should have known that one cannot obliterate any part of a life that has generally been so rich and so rewarding.

While I was writing, I found that even the old hurts and grievances gradually faded. I have moved on, focusing now on the way ahead rather than the road behind. I have indeed disposed of a weight off my mind.

APPENDIX

Weight Watchers first began in Datchet, Buckinghamshire. We had a banner on our house saying, 'WELCOME, PILGRIM — YOUR SEARCH IS ENDED'. And, indeed, our village became the centre of the Weight Watchers UK universe, a veritable Mecca to which devout members came from distant parts to seek inspiration and information. They visited my greengrocer to enquire what my family ate. At meetings, they asked me for specific ideas and recipes that I used myself. How did I entertain and still follow the Programme? How did I deal with binges? How did I make amends after cheating? But mostly they were interested in the foods and recipes that helped me with my particular crises. Although everyone's lifestyle is different, I have included some of those special recipes in this appendix for your enjoyment.

Soups & Appetisers

MID-MORNING BOUILLON
(SERVES 1)

8 fl oz/225 ml chicken stock made from bouillon cube
Dried garlic flakes or pressed garlic to taste
Few drops of lemon juice

Mix all the ingredients. Serve very hot. This bouillon is very refreshing on summer days served chilled.

BUTTON MUSHROOMS – WESTON STYLE

Merely place under grill until crisp and crunchy. Flavour with assorted spices and be heavy-handed with garlic salt or garlic.

CELERY AND FENNEL SOUP
(SERVES 2)

6 oz/175 g washed celery
Half a head of fennel
*½pt/300 ml water
*1 chicken stock cube
1 chopped onion
Salt and pepper
1 clove garlic
*Alternatively, use ½pt/300 ml of your own stock.

Cut the celery and fennel into small pieces. Place all the ingredients into a saucepan and bring to the boil. Simmer for 30 minutes then remove from heat, allow to cool slightly and liquidize.

CREAM OF CAULIFLOWER SOUP

Simmer cauliflower in good stock or water to which you have added a chicken stock cube. When tender, remove from heat and liquidize, adding a little skimmed milk from your allowance. This makes a very tasty 'free soup'.

COURGETTE CREOLE

Slice, without peeling, any amount of courgettes required. Place in saucepan. Pour over tomato juice from daily allowance. Season with garlic or garlic salt, pepper, minced parsley, bay leaf, pinch of basil, thyme. Cook over low flame to desired texture.

GOLDEN GRAPEFRUIT
(SERVES 2)

1 grapefruit, halved
Artificial sweetener to taste
1/4 teaspoon powdered cinnamon
Mint leaves to decorate

Pre-heat grill. Loosen flesh from sides of grapefruit and remove pips from centre. Mix together sweetener and cinnamon and spread over grapefruit halves. Grill for 4—5 minutes or until crisp and bubbly. Decorate with mint leaves.

HEART-WARMING SOUP
(SERVES 2)

8 fl oz/225 ml water
1 chicken stock cube   }   or 8 fl oz/225 ml stock
12 fl oz/350 ml tomato juice }
4 oz/100 g runner beans, fresh or frozen
4 oz/100 g mushrooms, sliced
2 teaspoons onion flakes or chopped onions
1 large chopped gherkin
1–2 teaspoons Worcester sauce
freshly ground black pepper

Place water, tomato juice and stock cube in saucepan, bring to boil. Add rest of ingredients and cook until tender (approximately 10–15 minutes). Serve piping hot or take to work in a Thermos flask.

HUNGARIAN THICK SOUP
(SERVES 4)

1 large tin celery hearts, drained
4 oz/100 g button mushrooms, sliced
½ pint/300 ml water
2 teaspoons paprika
¼ teaspoon dried tarragon
Salt and pepper

Liquidize the celery hearts or mash well with a fork. Place in a saucepan with the other ingredients. Bring to the boil, cover pan and simmer gently for 10–15 minutes. Adjust seasonings and serve.

TOMATO, ORANGE AND ONION SOUP
(SERVES 6)

2 teaspoons chopped onion or dried onion flakes,
    reconstituted
1 large can tomato juice
4 fl oz/100 ml low-cal orange squash
1 teaspoon cider vinegar
salt and black pepper

Combine all ingredients in saucepan and bring to the boil. Simmer until reduced and thickened. If there is any left over, this makes an excellent sauce for meat or fish.

WATERCRESS SOUP
(SERVES 1)

1 bunch watercress
½ pint/300 ml hot water
1 chicken stock cube
1 tablespoon skimmed milk
Ground black pepper

Wash watercress and roughly chop. Dissolve cube in hot water, add watercress and cook for 10 minutes. Remove from heat and liquidize. Add dried skimmed milk and reheat without bringing to the boil. Serve hot or well chilled, decorated with sprigs of watercress.

Main Courses and Accompaniments

CHEESE SOUFFLE
(SERVES 1)

4 fl oz/100 ml skimmed milk
1 egg, separated
1 oz/25 g cheddar cheese, grated
1 slice white bread, made into crumbs
1/8 teaspoon salt
Dash pepper

Combine milk, egg yolk, cheese and bread crumbs in a saucepan. Season with salt and pepper. Stir over a low heat until mixture is slightly thickened. Set aside to cool. Beat egg white until peaks form, fold into cooled mixture and put into soufflé dish. Bake at 190°C, 375°F, Mark 5, for 25 minutes.

CHICKEN MARENGO AND RICE
(SERVES 1)

8 oz/225 g chicken breast, thinly sliced and skinned
2 oz/50 g sliced onion
8 oz/225 g sliced mushrooms
1 chopped tomato
4 oz/100 g tomato juice
4 oz/100 g beef stock or stock cube and water
Dash garlic powder or pressed garlic
1/2 bay leaf

½ teaspoon Worcester sauce
Salt and pepper to taste
3 oz/75 g cooked rice

In a non-stick pan, slowly cook chicken for 5 minutes, remove and set aside. Place onions and mushrooms in the pan and cook until lightly brown. Add tomato, tomato juice, stock, garlic powder, bay leaf and Worcester sauce. Simmer 10 minutes or until mixture thickens. Season with salt and pepper. Place chicken in sauce and heat thoroughly. Serve over rice.

KILLARNEY IRISH STEW

8 oz/225 g lamb steak (boneless)
4 oz/100 g chopped onion (or 2 oz/50 g chopped leek and 2 oz/50 g onion)
1 stick celery, diced
1 medium (3 oz/75 g) potato, peeled and diced
⅛ teaspoon thyme
⅛ teaspoon rosemary
16 fl oz/350 ml chicken stock or stock cube and water
Salt and pepper to taste
1 teaspoon freshly chopped parsley

Grill lamb steak on rack, 4 in from heat about 5 minutes each side. Remove. Cool and cut into 1 in pieces. Place onions, celery and potato in saucepan. Add herbs and stock. Simmer for 20 minutes or until potatoes are tender. Add lamb, heat thoroughly. Season with salt and pepper. Sprinkle with parsley and serve.

NAVARIN OF VEAL

1 fillet of veal (6 oz/175 g)
1 cup of stock made with a cube

½ dessertspoon of raw chopped dried flaked onion,
    reconstituted
1 oz/25 g finely chopped celery
1 crushed garlic clove
1 cup tomato juice
2 oz/50 g chopped carrot
2 oz/50 g cooked french beans
Salt and pepper

Grill the veal on both sides until lightly cooked. Cut into
cubes and place in a non-stick pan along with the stock,
onion, celery and garlic. Simmer for 5 minutes. Add tomato
juice and carrots and cook for a further 5 minutes. Stir
green beans into the sauce, which will have reduced, and
cook until they have heated through. Serve at once. This
recipe serves one but can be adapted according to the
numbers you are cooking for.

SHEPHERD'S PIE
(SERVES 1)

6 oz/175 g minced lean cooked lamb
¼ pt/150 ml tomato juice
4 tablespoons beef stock or stock cube and water
1½ teaspoons chopped onion or reconstituted onion flakes
1½ teaspoons chopped pepper, red or green
1½ teaspoons chopped celery
Salt and pepper to taste
3 oz/75 g cooked potato
Paprika

Place the lamb in a saucepan with the tomato juice, stock,
onion, peppers, celery, herbs and seasoning. Bring to the
boil, stirring, cover pan and simmer for 15 minutes. Spoon
the mixture into an ovenproof dish. Mash the cooked
potato and place on top of the meat. Sprinkle with a little
paprika. Reheat in a hot oven (200°C, 400°F, Mark 6) for 15
minutes.

STUFFED MUSHROOMS FLORENTINE
(SERVES 1)

4 oz/100 g cooked spinach, finely chopped
2 oz/50 g cooked minced veal
1 slice white bread made into crumbs
¼ teaspoon garlic powder
2 teaspoons Worcester sauce
1 tablespoon freshly chopped parsley
1 teaspoon chopped onion or dried onion flakes,
    reconstituted in 1 tablespoon water
2 fl oz/50 ml liquid skimmed milk
salt and pepper to taste
8 oz/225 g large mushroom caps, stems removed
1 oz/25 g cheddar cheese, grated

Combine spinach, veal and bread crumbs in a mixing bowl. Add garlic powder, Worcester sauce, onion flakes and milk. Mix thoroughly until all liquid is absorbed. Season with salt and pepper. Fill mushroom caps with mixture and top with grated cheese. Bake on non-stick pan at 190°C, 375°F, Mark 5, for approximately 25 minutes or until cheese is bubbly.

SWEET AND SOUR CHICKEN

6 oz/175 g cooked chicken per person
Marinade: wine vinegar, salt, pepper, soy sauce, chilli sauce
            and/or Worcester sauce, sweetener, lemon juice.

Mix the marinade ingredients to taste. Place chicken in a large bowl and pour the marinade over the meat. Allow to stand for two to three hours. Transfer chicken and marinade into grill pan. Grill under low heat for 25–30 minutes, basting as required.

TOMATO FRENCH DRESSING

½ cup tomato juice
2 tablespoons vinegar
2 tablespoons chopped green pepper
½–1 teaspoon Worcester sauce
½ teaspoon salt
½ teaspoon dry mustard
1 clove pressed garlic or garlic salt to taste
¼ teaspoon liquid sweetener

Combine all ingredients in a blender and purée. Will keep in the fridge for a week.

Add horseradish for a combined dressing for salads or for prawns and other shellfish.

WEIGHT WATCHERS YORKSHIRE PUDDING
(SERVES 2)

2 eggs
2 oz/50 g white breadcrumbs
4 fl oz/100 ml skimmed milk
2 tablespoons cold water

Pre-heat oven to 230°C, 450°F, Mark 8. Combine all the ingredients in a liquidizer and run for 15 seconds. Sprinkle base of non-stick 7-inch baking tin with salt, pour in contents of liquidizer. Place on shelf near top of oven and bake until brown and well risen, approximately 20 minutes.

Cakes and Desserts

APPLE CREAM JELLY
(SERVES 1)

1 medium apple
Sweetener to taste
Few drops lemon juice
¼oz/7g skimmed milk powder
½ envelope of gelatine

Peel and slice apple. Sprinkle with lemon juice and place in a saucepan. Cover with water and simmer for 5 minutes. When cooked, place apple and juice in blender. Add sweetener, milk powder and gelatine and blend for 3 seconds.
   Place in dish and put in a cool place to set.

APPLE CRUMBLE
(SERVES 1)

1oz/25g white breadcrumbs
Grated peel of 1 lemon
1 medium-sized cooking apple, peeled and sliced
1 tablespoon lemon juice
Little artificial sweetener if necessary
3 slices of lemon, to decorate

Mix breadcrumbs and lemon rind together. Slowly cook apple in lemon juice in a covered pan until soft. Add a little artificial sweetener if necessary. Line a small individual pie dish with half of the breadcrumbs. Spoon in apple and cover with remaining breadcrumbs. Bake in a fairly hot oven (190°C, 375°F, Mark 5) for approximately 40 minutes, or until golden brown and crisp. Decorate with lemon slices.

APPLE QUEEN PUDDING
(SERVES 1)

5 tablespoons skimmed milk
Artificial sweetener to taste
1 slice bread, white, crumbed
1 egg
1 medium eating apple

Warm milk with 3 sweetener tablets. Pour over the crumbed bread and leave for 10 minutes. Separate egg and add yolk to bread mixture. Bake in a moderate oven (180°C, 350°F, Mark 4) for 15–20 minutes. Slice apple and stew with 4 tablespoons water and sweetener tablets. Pour over top of bread mixture and cover with stiffly beaten egg white (with 3 crushed sweetener tablets added) and bake for approximately 8 minutes in a fairly hot oven (200°C, 400°F, Mark 6).

BAKED APPLES STUFFED WITH RASPBERRIES
(SERVES 4)

4 medium cooking apples
8 oz/225 g fresh or frozen raspberries
¼ teaspoon cinnamon
Artificial sweetener to taste
¼ pint/150 ml water

Core the apples. Stand in shallow dish. Put water, sweetener and cinnamon into pan and bring to boil. Simmer one minute, then remove from the heat. Add whole raspberries and stuff centres of apples with this mixture. Pour remainder over top. Cover with foil and bake in centre of moderate oven (190°C, 350°F, Mark 4) for 25 minutes or until apples are tender.

CHOCOLATE CAKE BÉRÉNICE

4 eggs, separated
2 fl oz/50 ml water
6 teaspoons chocolate essence
¼ teaspoon artificial liquid sweetener
4 slices white bread, made into fine crumbs
1 oz/25 g skimmed milk powder

Chocolate icing:
2 oz/50 g low-fat spread
2 oz/50 g skimmed milk powder, sieved
¼ teaspoon artificial liquid sweetener
½ teaspoon vanilla essence
2 teaspoons chocolate essence

Preheat the oven to 180°C, 350°F, Mark 4. Place the egg yolks in a mixing bowl. Add the water, essence and artificial sweetener; whip until frothy. Add the breadcrumbs and skimmed milk powder and mix. Beat the egg whites until stiff peaks form. Carefully fold the egg whites into the yolk mixture and pour into a 7-inch square cake tin lined with greaseproof paper. Bake for about 25 minutes.

Slice in half, split each half in two. For the icing, combine the margarine, milk powder and sweetener. Slowly add the essence and mix. Chill and spread evenly between and on top of the cake. Mark the icing with a fork.

COFFEE LAYER CAKE
(SERVES 4)

4 eggs, separated
2 fl oz/50 ml water
4 teaspoons instant coffee powder
Sweetener to equal 10 teaspoons of sugar or to taste
4 slices enriched white bread made into fine crumbs
1 oz/25 g skimmed milk powder

Vanilla filling (see below)

Preheat oven to 180°C, 350°F, Mark 4. Place yolks in mixing bowl. Add water, coffee and sweetener. Whip until frothy. Add breadcrumbs and milk. Mix. Beat egg whites until stiff peaks form. Carefully fold whites into yolk mixture. Pour into a 9 in × 9 in tin, lined with non-stick baking paper. Bake for 30 minutes. Allow to cool. Peel off paper, slice cake in half horizontally and spread evenly with vanilla filling.

Vanilla Filling
4 tablespoons low-fat spread
1 oz/25 g skimmed milk powder
sweetener to taste
1 teaspoon vanilla extract OR 1 teaspoon instant coffee

Combine spread, milk and sweetener in a small bowl and mix with a wooden spoon. Slowly pour in extract and mix well. Chill and spread evenly between cake layers.

WEIGHT WATCHERS 'CREAM'

½ oz/12 g skimmed milk powder
½ teaspoon lemon juice
¼ teaspoon vanilla essence
½ fl oz/12 ml water
¼ teaspoon liquid sweetener

Combine all ingredients in a bowl and beat together until mixture stands in peaks.

GERMAN APPLE PANCAKE
(SERVES 1)

1 egg
2 tablespoons skimmed milk
sweetener to equal 3 tablespoons of sugar

¼ teaspoon cinnamon
1 slice white bread, made into crumbs
1 medium apple, peeled and grated

Preheat oven to 200°C, 400°F, Mark 6. Combine egg, milk, sweetener and cinnamon in mixing bowl. Add bread-crumbs and beat with hand whisk or fork for one minute. Pour into heated non-stick pan. Arrange apple on top. Immediately place in oven for 3–4 minutes until set. Remove, fold in half and serve.

ICY BANANA SHAKE
(SERVES 1)

1 ripe banana
½ pint/300 ml cold water
ice cubes
1 teaspoon cinnamon
½oz/12g dried skimmed milk, sweetened to taste with liquid
　　sweetener and made into thick paste with a little water
Pinch of salt

Mash the banana. Mix the water and sweetened milk, combining with the banana. Add the crushed ice cubes, cinnamon and salt. Beat until the mixture is smooth and ice cubes have melted. Serve immediately.

　　Instant coffee could be substituted or essence of chocolate, vanilla, brandy etc.

ORANGE DELIGHT
(SERVES 2)

1 large orange (peeled and cut into segments)
8 drops liquid sweetener
10 tablespoons skimmed milk

2 eggs, separated
2 drops vanilla essence

Beat the egg yolks with 4 drops of sweetener. Bring milk to boil and whisk in yolks and vanilla essence. Return to heat and cook very slowly, stirring all the time until mixture coats the back of a spoon. Do not boil. Pour sauce into 2 ovenproof dishes. Whisk egg whites with 4 drops sweetener, until stiff, the fold in chopped orange segments. Divide mixture between the 2 dishes and grill until brown.

PEAR NOIRE

1 pear
1 oz/25 g dried milk powder
1 cup of hot water
2 teaspoons of instant coffee

Peel the pear and poach in water until tender. Cut in half and remove core. Place on serving dish. Make up the coffee with the hot water, milk powder and sweetener, pour over the pear and serve hot or cold. (I prefer to use left-over coffee from the percolator for this dish, but instant will do if you make it nice and strong.)

PINEAPPLE SORBET

1 oz/25 g gelatine
4 slices fresh pineapple
4 dessertspoons fresh orange juice
juice of one lemon
liquid sweetener
pinch of ginger

Dissolve the gelatine with a little warm water, then place all the ingredients in a liquidizer and purée. Pour into a mould and leave in the fridge to set.

SUNSHINE ORANGE SOUFFLE
(SERVES 2)

7 fl oz/200 ml skimmed liquid milk
2 artificial sweetener tablets
2 medium oranges
2 slices bread, without crust
2 eggs, separated

Grate orange skins finely. Cut one slice from the middle of each orange — squeeze juice from ends, mix with grated rind and stir well. Heat milk with sweetener, but do not boil. Cut bread into small cubes and add to milk. Add orange juice and rind and continue stirring. Take off heat and add two beaten egg yolks. Quickly fold in stiffly beaten egg whites. Pour into a casserole dish. Place orange slices on top. Cook in a fairly hot oven (190°C, 375°F, Mark 5) for 5 minutes, then increase to 200°C, 400°F, Mark 6 for a further 20 or 25 minutes, or until golden brown and puffed.